POMEGRANATE
The Most Medicinal Fruit

ROBERT A. NEWMAN, PH.D.
AND EPHRAIM P. LANSKY, M.D.
WITH MELISSA LYNN BLOCK, M.ED.

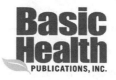

Basic Health
PUBLICATIONS, INC.

The information contained in this book is based upon the research and personal and professional experiences of the authors. It is not intended as a substitute for consulting with your physician or other healthcare provider. Any attempt to diagnose and treat an illness should be done under the direction of a healthcare professional.

The publisher does not advocate the use of any particular healthcare protocol but believes the information in this book should be available to the public. The publisher and authors are not responsible for any adverse effects or consequences resulting from the use of the suggestions, preparations, or procedures discussed in this book. Should the reader have any questions concerning the appropriateness of any procedures or preparation mentioned, the authors and the publisher strongly suggest consulting a professional healthcare advisor.

Basic Health Publications, Inc.
28812 Top of the World Drive
Laguna Beach, CA 92651
949-715-7327 • www.basichealthpub.com

Library of Congress Cataloging-in-Publication Data
Newman, Robert A., Ph. D.
  Pomegranate : the most medicinal fruit / Robert A. Newman,
Ephraim P. Lansky, with Melissa Lynn Block. — 1st ed.
    p. cm.
  Includes bibliographical references and index.
  ISBN 978-1-59120-210-3
1. Pomegranate—Health aspects. I. Lansky, Ephraim P. II. Block,
Melissa. III. Title.

  RM666.P798N49   2007
  615.8'54—dc22
                                            2007002926

Editor: Roberta W. Waddell
Copyeditor: John Anderson
Interior design and production: Gary A. Rosenberg
Cover design & illustration: Kris Waldherr

Printed in the United States of America

10   9   8   7   6   5   4   3   2   1

Contents

Acknowledgments

I am grateful to my co-authors, Robert A. Newman and Melissa Block, for their diligence, creativity, and quality control. Neal Holtzman and Steve Schwartz helped greatly to keep the process on track and the fires burning. Jarrow L. Rogovin and Peilin Guo were sources of inspiration. The following people assisted spiritually, materially, and energetically throughout: Drs. Shen Yu, Robert Zimmerman, and Martin Goldman, Edith, Zipora, Shifra, Yale, Aaron and Sidney Lansky, Cousin Barbara Mickelson, Ann Glassman, Matthew Robinson, Mark Efron, Yossi Diamant, Uri Burstyn, Eli Merom, Jacob Habooba, Shlomo Ben Shushan, and Rav Avidan Chazani.

—Ephraim P. Lansky

I would like to acknowledge the hard work and dedication of my co-authors and thank them for guiding me through this publishing experience. I am also truly grateful to our patients and their families, who are the driving force that inspires us on a daily basis to find and improve products of value for maintenance of good health and prevention of disease. To you, our valued reader: please know that a portion of the proceeds from the sale of this book are being used to develop the first pharmaceutical pomegranate product to one day directly assist in the prevention of breast cancer.

—Robert A. Newman

Thanks to Norman Goldfind for sending this fascinating project my way; to Ephraim Lansky for his commitment to integration of Nature's gifts with modern medicine; to Steve Schwartz and Neal Holtzman for their enthusiasm and patience; to Sue Emonds for her help and support; and to Bobby Waddell for her editorial expertise (and flexibility in the daunting face of Track Changes).

—Melissa Lynn Block

Introduction

The two of us, Robert A. Newman, Ph.D., and Ephraim P. Lansky, M.D., have been collaborating for years on the development of a botanical for use in the treatment and/or prevention of cancer. As a result of this search, we have found pomegranate to be an excellent candidate. We studied *in vitro* the effects of various components of this fruit—peel, seed, and juice—on the growth of breast, prostate, and skin cancer cells, and the results have been uniformly promising. We and fellow researchers have found that pomegranate is useful for other indications as well.

While research into creating specific pomegranate preparations is ongoing, pomegranate can be added to the diet in multiple ways *right now.* Juice, whole fruit, and supplements from properly prepared extracts can all provide benefits. Although our experience has been more in the realm of peer reviewed scientific journals, we decided to create this book about pomegranate's benefits to provide a bridge between the research and the public.

The pomegranate has long been used as a symbol of medicine. Patricia Langley's marvelous article, "Why a Pomegranate?", describes how the pomegranate has been held sacred by many of the world's major religions and how preparations of different parts of the plant have been used to treat a variety of

Royal College of Physicians Coat of Arms

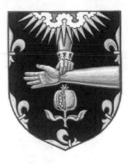

medical conditions through the ages. The pomegranate features in the coat of arms of several medical associations and it was chosen over DNA, the human body, and a heartbeat as the logo for the 2000 Millennium Festival of Medicine.

In Judaism, the pomegranate is a symbolic food representing sanctity, fertility, and abundance. Its seeds are said to number 613—one for each of the Bible's 613 commandments. The fruit has been featured in Jewish architecture and even decorated the pillars of King Solomon's temple. The *Song of Solomon* compares the cheeks of a bride behind her veil to the two halves of a pomegranate.

In Christian art, the pomegranate is a symbol of resurrection and eternal life. It is also found in paintings of the Virgin Mother and Child. In medieval representations, the pomegranate tree, a fertility symbol, is associated with the end of a unicorn hunt. According to legend, unicorns, wild by nature, can be tamed only by virgins. Once tamed, the unicorn was held in a garden and chained to a pomegranate tree, symbolizing the impending incarnation of Christ.

In her article, Langley describes the myth of the Greek goddess Persephone, in which the fruit has an integral part in the creation of the seasons. Persephone is allowed to travel from the underworld to the verdant surface of the Earth for a part of each year, bringing Spring and Summer to the planet, but she must return to the underworld each fall. Her union with Hades, the god of the underworld, is sealed not with a kiss, but with the consumption of a pomegranate seed.

Langley points out, "The pomegranate fruit is topped by a structure which provided the prototype for the crowns of kings;

the sanguine-colored juice brings to mind the life substance flowing through the arteries; and the multiplicity of seeds is a natural metaphor for reproductive success. These parallels suggested to the ancients that the pomegranate might also possess some impressive chemistry with direct practical relevance for the armamentarium of the physician. Contemporary medicine is beginning to recognize this as well. The pomegranate enjoys a coveted medicinal image with multi-faceted applications for protection and improvement of health."

This guide to the pomegranate details what each part of the fruit—seeds, juice, and peel—has to offer. Even the tree's leaves, bark, and roots have therapeutic properties. This venerable fruit is filled with much more than just juicy red seeds, known as arils. (*Wikipedia* defines an aril as "a fleshy covering of certain seeds formed from the funinculus, the attachment point of the seed.")

Chapter 1 provides an overview of the chemical composition and history of the pomegranate.

Chapter 2 proposes that pomegranate deserves a place in the realm of superfoods, delivering numerous potent health benefits.

Chapter 3 details how pomegranate affects women's health, including breast cancer and osteoporosis. The fruit also has properties that aid in protecting postmenopausal women against heart disease.

Chapter 4 discusses how men may benefit from the pomegranate, with research showing that the fruit attacks prostate cancer cells and protects prostate health.

Chapter 5 elaborates on pomegranate as a heart-healthy food, thanks to its rich stores of antioxidants that help reduce the risk of atherosclerosis, high cholesterol, hypertension, and ischemic heart disease.

Chapter 6 addresses pomegranate's salutary effects on metabolism, which can benefit those with diabetes, insulin resistance, metabolic syndrome, or obesity.

Chapter 7 delves into how pomegranate seed oil may benefit the skin. Its anti-inflammatory properties can provide quick relief from minor skin irritations. No small wonder that pomegranate seed oil is turning up in many skincare products today.

Chapter 8 contains our recommendations for what features to look for in a pomegranate dietary supplement, juice, or juice concentrate.

Chapter 9 discusses our plans for future development of pomegranate compounds.

We offer this book in the belief that the more that is learned about pomegranate's many benefits, the more people will want to include this remarkable fruit in their diets and supplements.

A Wealth of Phytochemicals

ategorized as a berry, the pomegranate is a handsome fruit. It holds many small fruits—or *arils*—wrapped tightly inside a leathery, red rind.

Unlike other plants, the pomegranate belongs to its own botanical family—Punicaceae—with only one genus—*Punica*—and one predominant species—*P. granatum*. A second species of *Punica* does exist, a smaller and more primitive version of the tree. Unfortunately, this rare type occurs only on the isolated island of Socotra, off the cost of Yemen. Like the Galapagos, Socotra is home to many species which exist only on these islands.

POMEGRANATE	
Order: Myrtales	Genus: *Punica*
Family: Punicaceae	Species: *P. granatum*

The Whole Plant

The pomegranate tree is long-lived, with some European trees living over 200 years though fruit production declines after about fifteen years. The trees are rounded and shrub-like, yet can grow to thirty feet in height; they do not usually grow beyond twelve to sixteen feet. Dwarf varieties are available. The tree's bark is reddish-brown when the plant is young and later matures to a grayish tone. Depending on where the tree grows, it may retain or lose its glossy, thick, narrow, and pointed leaves seasonally. Fruit may be produced within a few months of planting, or it may not appear for up to three years. Hot temperature during the fruiting period yields the sweetest fruits.

The Flower

Pomegranate flowers are usually orange, though red, pink, or white flowers have also been described. They are an inch or more in diameter, and their red fleshy *calyx,* the crown-like protuberance at the fruit's base, is the first sign of the fruit to come. Insects are required for thorough pollination, but the flowers can also self-pollinate.

Whole Fruit

Each fruit can be from two-and-a-half to five inches in diameter. The calyx is prominent, and the leathery rind may be yellow, deep pink, red, or even a deep, glowing rubine red such as those from Israel's Galilee. The size can vary from a large apple weighing 200 grams to the size and shape of a small rugby ball weighing 700–900 grams. Those grown in the Galilee of northern Israel are largest.

Arils/Seeds

When you cut open a pomegranate in anticipation of eating the fruit, the arils—the juice encapsulated seeds—are what you're after. The arils nest, the interior of the fruit, is divided into many chambers. Be sure to open your pomegranate in a place where it's acceptable to make a bit of a mess. Use a plate at least as large as a dinner plate and be sure not to wear anything that you'll regret staining as you're cutting up a fruit.

Biting into a pomegranate aril is a curious and pleasurable experience. It bursts in your mouth with a tart-sweet, ripe, juicy crunchiness. Jewish lore states that the fruit contains 613 arils, one for each commandment in the Five Books of Moses, but botanists note anywhere from 200 to more than 800 are found, depending on the size of the fruit.

About 18 percent dry weight of the cleaned, white seeds (found inside the juicy, translucent arils) is oil. Once the juice is removed from the arils, an oil rich in punicic acid can be extracted from the seeds, which can then be used as a skincare aid. The remainder of the seed, known as seed cake, contains a matrix of lignins and polysaccharides that comprise the cell walls. In this matrix, other physiologically potent compounds are found. All these aspects of the fruit are being investigated for their health benefits.

FATTY ACIDS

The basic building blocks of fats and oils; made of long chains of carbon molecules bound by single, double, or triple bonds in various configurations.

Punicic acid is a triple conjugated 18-carbon fatty acid that makes up 65 percent of the volume of pomegranate seed oil. Conjugated, in the case of punicic acid, means that it has within its 18-carbon chain three different double bonds, between carbons 5 and 6, 7 and 8, and 9 and 10. Between carbons 6 and 7 and between carbons 8 and 9 are single bonds, and this alternation between double and single bonds is what makes these fatty acids conjugated.

Conjugated fatty acids with two alternating double bonds, as opposed to three, are called conjugated linoleic acids (CLA). CLAs are found in the milk and meat of ruminant animals, such

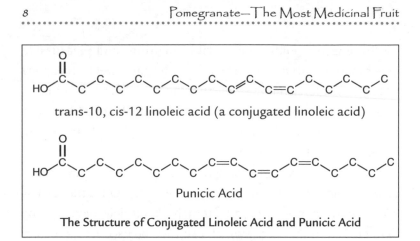

trans-10, cis-12 linoleic acid (a conjugated linoleic acid)

Punicic Acid

The Structure of Conjugated Linoleic Acid and Punicic Acid

as cattle and sheep. Ordinary linoleic acid, an essential fatty acid, is also abundant in pomegranate seed oil, comprising about 10 percent of the oil by weight.

LIGNINS
Highly hydrophobic components of cell walls useful for tensile strength and transportation of water within the plant. Subcomponents of lignins, including lignans, provide antioxidant, anti-cancer, and estrogenic effects.

POLYSACCHARIDES
A type of complex or long chain carbohydrate.

Scientific research has shown that the physiologically potent compounds found in seed cake are used by the plant for regulating its own physiology. Many of those compounds happen to be similar to substances well known in human physiology, including sex steroid hormones.

Mammalian estrogens were discovered before phytoestrogen—a plant compound producing estrogenic effects in the bodies of animals, including humans—became a household word. Today, most references to phytoestrogens in the popular media refer primarily to isoflavones found in soy and the lignans in flax, but the pomegranate's phytoestrogenic properties are just as impressive, perhaps even more so. Some of the phytoestrogen compounds found in pomegranate are minute amounts of real steroid hormones, such as estriol, estrone, and even testosterone. In our own investigations, we also discovered a large store of 17-alpha-estradiol in pomegranate seed oil. This compound is a mirror-image version of the estrogen produced in the highest quantities in the female body. To the best of our knowledge, this was the first time it had ever been found in a plant source.

SEX STEROID HORMONE

Any hormone made from cholesterol that controls sexuality and reproduction; includes estrogens (estradiol, estriol, estrone), progesterone, and testosterone. Sex steroids also have global effects on the health of bone, skin, cardiovascular system, and other internal organs.

Juice

As with all fruit juices, pomegranate juice has its share of natural sugars (fructose, glucose, and sucrose) and simple organic acids (ascorbic, citric, fumaric, malic). The juice even contains small amounts of all the essential amino acids (protein building blocks) and of these, it is richest in proline (the precursor of cartilage), methionine (a sulphur-containing amino acid that has antioxidant activities), and valine (a branched-chain amino acid).

BRANCHED-CHAIN AMINO ACIDS

A class of unique protein building blocks essential for life. Supplements are popular with athletes because they are said to aid in steady energy production.

Peel

Although the fruit's peel is tough and unappetizing, its bitterness means it is rich in compounds with potential therapeutic uses. Most of the important pharmacological activity of the peel and juice both come from a broad class of compounds called *polyphenols*. These include *tannins* and *flavonoids*, which are natural preservatives and powerful antioxidants.

Antioxidant Polyphenols Also Protect Against the Hazards of Obesity

Certain naturally occurring phytochemicals found in plants can decrease insulin resistance. Promising research finds that, in some cases, these plant chemicals can restore appropriate balance in insulin-resistant people.

One class of phytochemicals that can normalize the insulin resistance underlying metabolic conditions is the polyphenols. These polyphenols are found in pomegranate juice, peels, and seed oil.

Most of the important activity of the juice, as well as the peels, comes from this broad class of compounds called polyphenols. To understand the basic concept of what a polyphenol is, it is important to first become acquainted with two structures: the benzene ring and phenol.

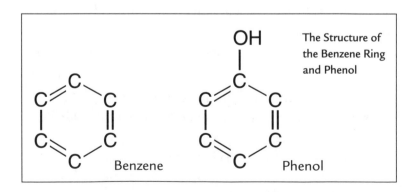

The Structure of the Benzene Ring and Phenol

Benzene

Phenol

Simply, the benzene ring is a hexagonal shape consisting of six carbon atoms. Whenever you see the familiar hexagons in complex chemical drawings, they are usually these benzene rings; they recur as a pattern in many organic compounds. The original idea for the benzene ring to explain the observed phenomenon of the molecules in this configuration came to the chemist Freidrich Kekule (1829–1896) as a dream of a serpent biting its own tail—the mythical *ourobouros*.

A phenol is a benzene ring with one hydroxyl group—an oxygen and a hydrogen (OH) bound together—attached to one of the carbons. Polyphenols refer to complexes built up from more than one of these phenols.

The benzene ring (like its derivatives) is an example of a *conjugated* system, where double and single bonds alternate along the carbon chain. The benzene ring is also an aromatic system, meaning that electrons are passed off from one carbon to the other, in effect constantly moving the double bonds from one position on the ring to the next. In other words, the molecule is in a constant state of flux. As with the conjugated fatty acids described above, this makes polyphenols biologically highly active.

The polyphenols come in many chemical forms, but the two largest classes relevant to pomegranate juice are tannins and flavonoids. They are natural preservatives and powerful antioxidants.

One type of tannin, called an *ellagitannin,* breaks down into hydroxybenzoic acids, such as ellagic acid. This very powerful antioxidant prevents skin flaps from dying during plastic surgery. Punicalagin and punicalin are specific ellagitannins found in both pomegranate peel and pomegranate juice.

Flavonoids are another form of polyphenol that share a particular chemical structure called the flavan nucleus. Several classes of flavonoids are found in pomegranate, including anthocyanins, flavan-3-ols, flavonols, and flavones. Flavan-3-ols include catechins, most often thought of as beneficial components of green tea.

Catechins are powerful antioxidants which are also found in pomegranate peel and juice. They are the building blocks of proanthocyanidins, also powerful antioxidants and the progenitors of anthocyanins, yet another class of antioxidant/anti-inflammatory compounds.

Anthocyanins are found mainly in the juice, not the peel, and are responsible for the juice's bright red color. They are also antioxidants, but unlike the tannins, flavonols, and flavones, are themselves very easily broken down by oxidation. In fermented pomegranate juice, the flavonoids are particularly bioavailable and active. All these are potent antioxidants, which also have the indirect effect of inhibiting certain compounds that accelerate inflammation, such as tumor necrosis factor (TNF-*alpha*).

Bark and Roots

The bark and roots of the pomegranate tree contain chemicals called *alkaloids*. These complex carbon-based compounds, which also include the element nitrogen, possess numerous potent physiological effects. Some examples of herbs possessing useful alkaloids include barberry, cacao, goldenseal, Oregon grape, poppy, and turmeric. Alkaloids found in the roots and bark of the pomegranate tree have been used for centuries in traditional medicine against worms that inhabit the human gastrointestinal tract.

Nutritional Information

One raw, 200 gram pomegranate contains:

- 105 calories

- 1.46 grams of protein

- 26.4 grams of carbohydrates

- 0.46 grams of total fat

- 5 grams of fiber if you eat the seeds, less than one gram if you don't

- 9.4 milligrams of vitamin C—15 percent of the U.S. RDA

History and Geography

The pomegranate's story meanders around the globe and through the millennia. For thousands of years, many cultures have believed in the various benefits of the pomegranate for health, fertility, longevity, and rebirth.

Though cultivated in the United States today (especially Central California), the pomegranate is native to the Middle East and was later grown in the Mediterranean. It grows well in semi-arid, mild-temperate to subtropical climates, where the air is dry, summers are hot, and winters are cool but not colder than 12° Fahrenheit (−11° Centigrade). Pomegranate trees can be grown in containers in greenhouses.

Pomegranates are mentioned in the Bible and appear in Greek mythology. For centuries, they have been hallowed throughout Asia, alongside the grape and the fig. In fact, the pomegranate has countless claims to fame.

- Babylonians believed that chewing pomegranate seeds before entering combat made them invincible.

- Ancient Egyptians buried their rulers with pomegranates.

- Pomegranate designs were used to decorate the garb of high priests in the first and second temples in Jerusalem.

- The pomegranate is one of the three blessed fruits in Buddhism, along with the citrus and the peach. In one legend, an

evil child-eating goddess was cured of her habit when the
Buddha gave her a pomegranate to eat. She became a symbol
of fertility, and today, Japanese Buddhist women may be
instructed to pray to this goddess if they have trouble con-
ceiving a child.

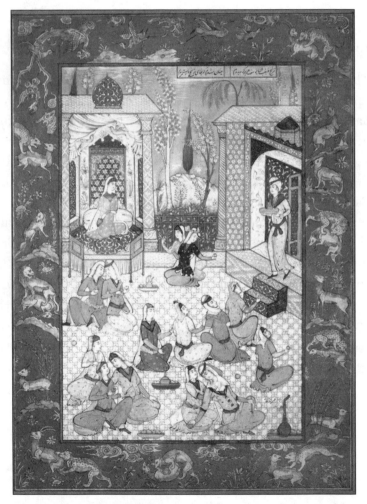

Persian painting depicting Biblical scene of Joseph entering court of the
wife of Potiphar, the chamberlain and captain of the Pharaoh's guard.
The courtesans are slicing pomegranates and are taken by Joseph's beauty.

- In the famed *Song of Solomon,* the blushing cheeks of a bride are compared to the two halves of a pomegranate.

- The pomegranate was the official emblem of Holy Roman Emperor Maximilian I.

- Devotional Christian art often features the pomegranate as a symbol of resurrection and eternal life.

- Granada, a city in Spain, and Grenada, an island in the Lesser Antilles of the Caribbean, were named after the Spanish and French word for pomegranate.

- A popular wedding present in Chinese culture is a picture of a split pomegranate. Among Bedouins in the Middle East, a new bridegroom splits a ripe pomegranate as he and his new wife enter their dwelling. If the fruit has many seeds and the bride and groom eat them, they are said to be promised many children.

- To bring abundance, fertility, and good luck to anyone who purchases a new home in Greece, house guests bring a pomegranate on their first visit.

Today, the evidence in favor of the pomegranate's legendary health benefits has caused Americans to take notice. With a healthy supply of antioxidants, the power to reduce inflammation, the ability to help regulate hormones in menopausal women, and a host of other benefits, the pomegranate has become a hot commodity.

Popularization of Pomegranate

According to a 2005 AC Nielsen study, United States sales of pomegranate juice have grown from $84,507 in 2001 to a whopping $66,240,767 in 2005. You can now buy the juice bottled, fresh, or concentrated. Pomegranate is available in various forms for the health-conscious consumer:

- Powdered capsules and tablets, which can contain the seed, fermented juice, peel, leaf, and/or flower

- Seed oil extracts, both bottled and in soft gelatin capsules

- Tea, brewed by the manufacturer from pomegranate leaves or seeds and packaged as a beverage, or available as a dry herbal tea

- Food and beverage products containing pomegranate, such as jams and jellies, salad dressings, sauces, and vinegars

- Dried pomegranate seeds, known as *anardana,* sometimes ground into a powder for use as a spice, and typically used in Indian, Iranian, and Pakistani cooking

- And, of course, the whole fruit

Practical Tips and Recipes contains lots of good information on how to integrate pomegranate into your daily life.

HONORABLE MENTION
The U.S. Centers for Disease Control and Prevention honored the pomegranate with "Fruit of the Month" status in September 2005.

2

A Pleiotrope by
Any Other Name

Pleiotrope refers to any product affecting multiple changes. We use the word here in the sense of a medicine that affects multiple phyisiological improvements. (In medicine, *pleiotrope* generally refers to a genetic change which affects a wide range of physiological alterations.)

Since Ayurveda of India, one of the oldest medical systems, considers the pomegranate to be a "pharmacy unto itself," pleiotrope is a suitable word to apply to the pomegranate. According to Ayurvedic medicine, the juice is a powerful aid in lowering fevers, its bright red color reflecting its reputation as a blood tonic. In ancient Greek medicine, pomegranate flowers were regarded as a treatment for diabetes. Even the roots and bark of the tree were used to treat infections caused by worms and related parasites. The leather-like peels of the fruits are boiled by folk healers around the world into tannin-rich potions used to staunch bleeding, check dysentery, and heal ulcers.

By the sixteenth century, the Royal College of Medicine in Great Britain had already assigned the pomegranate a spot in its coat of arms. This fruit's medicinal value has been appreciated as far back as ancient Greece, during which time—again, according to Langley's article—famed physician Dioscorides wrote: "All sorts of pomegranates are of a pleasant taste and good for your stomach . . . the juice of the kernels pressed out, being . . . mixed with honey, are good for the ulcers that are in your mouth and in your genitals . . . also for . . . ulcers, pains of the ears, and for . . . griefs in the nostrils . . . decoction of the flowers [helps] moist flagging gums and loose teeth . . . the rind having a binding faculty . . . decoction of the roots doth expel and kill [parasites]." Although knowledge about the pomegranate is more scientific today, Dioscorides was unquestionably right about many of pomegranate's healing effects.

Assignation as symbol of the British Millennial Festival of Medicine notwithstanding, the pomegranate had been all but forgotten as a serious source of health benefits in both the modern East and West. This appears to be on the verge of changing because research published in the past eight years is supporting ancient reports about pomegranate juice, peels, flowers, and seed oil.

Today, we understand more than ever before about *why* pomegranate has so many beneficial health effects. These appear to be largely attributable to chemical constituents of the fruit that promote or help to restore what we believe is a basically healthful balance at the body's cellular level. Although their actions and properties are complex, we can reduce them to two common denominators: antioxidant and anti-inflammatory effects.

Throughout this book, you will find references to and fuller explanations of these two common denominators, which are now believed to be important causative and accelerating factors in aging and health. The complex anti-inflammatory effects of pomegranate are a recent discovery, although research has long extolled the pomegranate's rich chemistry for its potent antioxidant activities. This fruit is said to have a higher concentration of antioxidant factors than any other besides the acai, a rainforest fruit that is far less palatable.

As fruits go, pomegranate is enormously complicated, with a

great many parts and chemical constituents. Once you've gotten to know these well, we'll return to the question of how this fruit—technically a berry—lives up to the high expectations you might have of a symbol of medicine.

> **ANTIOXIDANT**
> A substance that helps neutralize free radicals
> that attack cells.

The main argument in favor of considering pomegranate to be a pleiotrope has to do with its effects on a process that, in recent years, has been identified as a sort of common denominator of most of the health problems Westerners face.

Common Causes, Common Cures— A New, Old Medical Question

The diseases that most commonly affect people today are not the types of diseases that once caused most death and debility. In modern countries, there appears less fear of infection or trauma because they are generally responsive to current, advanced medicine. Today's biggest challenges are of a different sort: allergies, arthritis, asthma, autoimmune diseases, cancer, diabetes, heart disease, hormone imbalances, infertility, and other disease states that tend to be caused by multiple, interwoven factors, and are chronic and difficult to treat with drugs or surgery.

> **CHRONIC DISEASE**
> A disease that may be controlled through medical means,
> but does not have a medical cure—a disease which can
> persist over many years.

Chronic diseases, which more often seem to spring from a combination of genetic susceptibility and imbalances in diet and lifestyle habits, require a more general approach. However, knowledge does run in cycles. Today, a "new" undercurrent that originated in the oldest forms of medicine seems to be pointing *to common streams of causation—**and, accordingly,** to common sources of treatment.* These common factors include inflammation and oxidation.

The Role of Inflammation

Inflammation is the body's natural healing response to injury but it is also a common cause of disease. These are four cardinal signs of inflammation: redness, swelling, heat, and pain.

These signs are all symptoms of a cascade of events whereby boundaries break down in the tissues and lymph fluid and blood move in to effect repair. The fluids are full of white blood cells (lymphocytes) which can destroy pathogenic (harmful) cells and repair injuries.

Other body chemicals known as *cytokines* amplify the inflammatory process and further the mechanisms of repair. Still other compounds, *matrix metalloproteinases,* are primarily responsible for disrupting the integrity of tissues and the walls of blood vessels. This allows the fluids of inflammation to flow into areas where repair is needed.

Inflammation can be triggered by tissue damage, ultraviolet radiation from the sun, mechanical trauma, or infection by bacteria and viruses. Microscopic injury to the interior of arteries can lead to a buildup of inflammation that, in turn, leads to the creation of plaques in the vessels that feed the heart muscle and brain, increasing susceptibility to heart attacks and strokes.

Inflammation can also arise in an *autoimmune* form, where the immune system creates inflammation that isn't needed to keep the body safe, but actually attacks and damages healthy tis-

Inflammation and Oxidation

Inflammation is mediated by several of the body's physiologic systems, including the immune and endocrine (hormonal) systems. One system of special interest involves the production and action of the *eicosanoids,* bioactive molecules that are produced in the cells from the fats people eat. The eicosanoids are a class of hormone-like chemicals that includes the subclasses *prostaglandins* and *leukotrienes.* As it turns out, the pomegranate has several salutary effects on the balance of these chemicals (more on this to come).

Oxidation is a natural process that occurs as each cell creates energy from fuel (carbohydrates and fats). As energy is made, byproducts—*free radicals*—are formed. As with inflammation, this natural process can become unbalanced, and this imbalance can lead to damage in cell membranes and DNA, predisposing people to arthritis, cancer, and coronary artery disease.

Inflammation and oxidation tend to exacerbate each other.

sues. Allergies, asthma, Crohn's disease, eczema, lupus, psoriasis, and rheumatoid arthritis are all examples of autoimmune inflammation.

Although inflammation is essential for repair of acute problems, *the real trouble begins when it continues as a chronic, unresolved process.* It's like a fire alarm going off and then continuing to sound long after the initial blaze has been quelled. Destruction is then wrought by the inflammatory process itself as a cycle that just keeps on going.

Chronic inflammation causes the body to stay fixed in an emergency mode. One consequence is that certain steroid hormones, produced abundantly during stressful times, begin to influence the body even more powerfully than insulin, the hormone produced by the pancreas to move blood sugars into body cells for use as energy. In certain states of inflammation and stress, insulin pours out of the pancreas but the hormone has little or no effect. Blood sugar and insulin levels become chronically high, and both collaborate to damage blood vessels, nerves, and vital organs. *Insulin resistance* (IR) is the name of this condition. It has become common and turns into type 2 diabetes once the pancreas becomes too exhausted to make enough insulin to move sugars into cells.

Problems that spring from insulin resistance account for much more than diabetes. IR predisposes one to abdominal obesity, atherosclerosis (a buildup of plaques in the arteries of the heart), dyslipidemia (elevated LDL cholesterol and triglycerides), heart disease, and deposits of *amyloid* proteins in the brain, hallmarks of dementia and Alzheimer's disease. The original name for this collection of insulin- and blood sugar–related symptoms is *syndrome X,* but it is mainly referred to now as *metabolic syndrome.*

Depression, polycystic ovary syndrome (PCOS), and cancer can also spring from chronic inflammation. Inflammation can also lodge itself in specific tissues, causing arthritis, inflammatory bowel syndrome, and ulcers.

Pomegranate, Eicosanoids, and Inflammation

In the laboratory of the late Professor Ishak Neeman at the Technion-Israel Institute of Technology in Haifa, Israel, a study was conceived to determine just how effective pomegranate fractions were at addressing these two common denominators of disease—inflammation and oxidation. Schubert, Lansky, and Neeman used fermented pomegranate juice and cold-pressed seed oil in their study, and found that both of these fractions had antioxidant efficacy close to that of green tea and the widely used antioxidant preservative butylated hydroxyanisole (BHA). The fermented juice and seed oil both had antioxidant activity significantly greater than that of red wine. A pomegranate fraction inhibited the cyclooxygenase (COX-2) enzyme by 31–44 percent, by any measure, a significant anti-inflammatory effect.

Fermented Juice

Why fermented pomegranate juice? Fermentation is the process by which grapes are made into wine, soy is made into tempeh or miso, cabbage is made into sauerkraut, apple cider is made into vinegar, and milk is made into yogurt. Fermentation describes the action of specific bacteria or yeasts on food, transforming it—often into a more bioavailable and health-enhancing form. Humans have been fermenting foods since the dawn of time, and research strongly suggests it is beneficial to human health. Dr. Lansky has found in his various investigations of the pomegranate that fermented juice is often superior in its effects to fresh juice. The beneficial compounds of pomegranate juice are bound to sugars that must be digested before absorption of the nutrients can occur. When the juice is fermented, the polyphenol-sugar bonds are naturally broken via a process known as zymolysis. When tested, fermented pomegranate juice (with the alcohol removed) is a far more potent antioxidant source than is fresh pomegranate juice.

Oxidation—Sparks from the Fire of Metabolism

In addition to serving as a necessary basis of life in the air we breathe, oxygen can also have a damaging effect on the body. The normal process of cellular metabolism—the production of energy from the breakdown of carbohydrates and fats in the diet—naturally produces highly reactive byproducts called *free radicals.* At its most basic level, a free radical is an unbalanced, chemically reactive molecule that is missing one electron. Electrons like to travel in pairs, and in the process of metabolism, electron pairs are split in half.

The molecule with the single electron becomes a magnet for other single electrons. It starts to steal electrons from other molecules—fats, proteins, DNA. Free radicals seek electrons to make intact pairs. A free radical is, in essence, a molecular toxin—it takes for itself another electron pair, oxidizing the other molecule or even turning it into a free radical. The new free radical goes hunting for single electrons to satisfy its own quest for balance. Eventually, if left unchecked, this chain of events can disrupt a cell's normal functioning, leading to cell destruction and tissue damage.

Oxidation can cause damage on its own and it can act to promote inflammation. The body responds to this assault with inflammation in all its many guises. Oxidation and inflammation feed each other, forming an escalating cycle that causes aging and harms the body when not adequately controlled.

Antioxidants are the body's natural defense against these destructive oxygen free radicals. Some antioxidants prevent the damage from starting; others stop the damage while it is occurring; still others facilitate repair after the damage has occurred. Pomegranates are one of the most abundant storehouses of antioxidant nutrients known to contemporary nutritional science.

The Role of Metabolic Syndrome

Metabolic syndrome is a constellation of conditions that predisposes the body to accelerated inflammation *and* oxidation. It ages the body more rapidly and increases vulnerability to heart disease and some cancers. It has become increasingly common, affecting some 50 million individuals in America alone.

Metabolic syndrome, which is often a precursor to type 2 diabetes, is characterized by:

- Abdominal obesity, where fat accumulates in the abdominal area.

- Dyslipidemia, where LDL cholesterol and triglycerides are high and HDL cholesterol is low.

- High blood pressure (hypertension).

- Insulin resistance, where cells become less responsive to insulin. As a result, blood sugars rise along with insulin levels as the pancreas tries to overcome the cells' insulin resistance. Elevated insulin increases inflammation, oxidation, and *glycation,* the complexing of sugars to proteins such as hemoglobin. Glycation damages eye tissue and decreases the youthful resilience of body tissues, and that, itself, accelerates inflammation and oxidation even further.

- A prothrombic state, where the blood becomes more prone to clotting because the platelets, which are responsible for normal clotting, become too "sticky"—increasing the risk of clots and stroke.

- A pro-inflammatory state elevating markers of whole-body inflammation such as *C-reactive protein* (CRP).

The metabolic syndrome is bad news for the circulatory system. It dramatically increases the likelihood of heart attack or occlusive stroke, where a clot or a constricted vessel slows or halts the flow of blood to the heart muscle or to parts of the brain. Studies of the various factors of this syndrome have helped scientists understand how inflammation and oxidation are both key players in the development of heart disease, which remains the number-one killer of adult men and women in the United States and other Western nations. It will come as no surprise that aspects of the pomegranate, effective against inflammatory/oxidative damage, show promise in improving health and longevity.

Pomegranate Cools the Fires of Inflammation and Oxidation

Pomegranate counters both the oxidative and the inflammatory aspects of this cycle, being one of Nature's most abundant sources of antioxidants and containing anti-inflammatory phytochemicals (plant chemicals). Below are some specific ways in which pomegranates fight inflammation and oxidation.

- Pomegranate juice and peels contain potent antioxidants that help contain the inflammatory/oxidant cascade from spiraling beyond what's needed for healing.

- Pomegranate juice and peel extracts interfere with inflammatory cytokines and key transcription factor *NF-kappa Beta.*

- A unique fatty acid, *punicic acid,* is found in pomegranate seed oil; this fat inhibits the formation of inflammatory prostaglandins and other eicosanoids.

- Pomegranate extracts have been found to inhibit the oxidation of LDL cholesterol (the bad cholesterol) a pivotal event in the cascade that leads to atherosclerosis (buildup of plaques in coronary arteries). Pomegranate juice has been shown to enhance the production of a substance in the artery wall that relaxes vessels, improving blood flow.

- A study performed at Case Western University, published in the September 2005 edition of the *Journal of Nutrition,* found that pomegranate fruit extracts reduce the activity of a pro-inflammatory protein, *interleukin-1b,* believed to play a key role in the cartilage degradation caused by osteoarthritis.

- Pomegranate flowers are rich in a class of compounds called *triterpenoids,* which can nudge cells to show more sensitivity to insulin.

- Pomegranate extracts are being investigated as chemopreventive agents to prevent, slow, or halt the growth of cancerous cells; they show particular promise against prostate and breast cancers. It is believed that the anti-inflammatory, antioxidant effects of pomegranate phytochemicals are, at least in part, responsible for these chemopreventive effects.

In short, pomegranate seems to possess within its seeds, flowers, peels, and juice the chemical wherewithal to turn the tides of chronic inflammation, stem the destruction of metabolic syndrome, and help bring cellular events back to normal.

Osteoarthritis

Research suggests that the pomegranate can help relieve the pain and debility of the over 20 million Americans who have osteoarthritis. This degenerative disease is associated with a breakdown of cartilage in the joints, and can occur in almost any joint in the body, especially the hips, knees, and spine.

Cartilage is the hard, resilient, slippery coating on the ends of the bones that allows bone ends to slide smoothly past each other. When cartilage breaks down, the exposed bone can then break down, causing pain, inflammation, and disability. Though most people over the age of sixty have some degree of osteoarthritis, the phenomenon can strike people in their twenties and thirties as well.

Numerous factors influence a person's chances of developing osteoarthritis: heredity, injury, lack of activity, obesity, and overuse. Symptoms of osteoarthritis typically develop gradually and include joint soreness, especially with movement; joint swelling; bony enlargements in the middle and end joints of the fingers; and pain after long periods of inactivity or after excessive use.

Treatment often does almost nothing to actually *treat* the disease. People with osteoarthritis can often do little more than try to control pain with acetaminophen or NSAIDs, and those who use the latter class of drugs can develop gastrointestinal bleeding. A new study, however, shows that pomegranate fruit extract might help reduce the need for medicines by slowing the deterioration of cartilage associated with osteoarthritis.

Researchers studied the ability of pomegranate to inhibit the activity of interleukin-1b, an inflammatory protein molecule that plays a role in cartilage degradation. In a 2005 Case Western Reserve University School of Medicine study published in the *Journal of Nutrition,* scientists found that pomegranate extract slowed down the deterioration of human cartilage by reducing levels of the destructive interleukin-1b protein, and by suppressing enzymes that cause cartilage deterioration.

It probably comes as no surprise that inflammation and oxidation play roles in accelerating the degradation of cartilage in people with arthritis. Consumption of pomegranate fruit—with its antioxidant and anti-inflammatory properties—may inhibit cartilage deterioration in osteoarthritis, and may also be useful for maintaining joint integrity and function in those without the disease.

Boosting the Effectiveness of Antibiotics

Antibiotics have saved the lives of millions, perhaps billions, of people who, before their discovery, might have been felled by infectious diseases that now raise little concern. Yet the extensive, widespread use of these drugs has raised the specter of antibiotic resistance, where bacteria morph into strains that can't be controlled by conventional antibiotic therapy.

A study published in the *Canadian Journal of Microbiology* has shed light on a lesser-known potential use for pomegranate as an antibiotic booster. Researchers found a synergistic interaction between concentrated pomegranate extract and antibiotics in killing off antibiotic-resistant strains of *Staphylococcus aureus.* According to the study's authors, when pomegranate extract was tested against this dangerous microorganism, alongside five different antibiotics—ampicillin, chloramphenicol, gentamicin, oxacillin, and tetracycline—it "dramatically enhanced the activity of all antibiotics tested . . . and thus, offers an alternative for the extension of the useful lifetime of these antibiotics."

> **SYNERGY**
> The interaction of two or more agents or forces so their combined effect is greater than the sum of their individual effects.

Pomegranate, the "Anti"-Fruit

Pomegranate compounds possess antibacterial and antiviral activity. The rind of the pomegranate is known to have both antiviral and antifungal qualities, and the leaves have long been used in folk medicine as antibacterial topical wound dressings. The antioxidant polyphenols in the pomegranate take down free-radical scavengers resulting from oxidation. And where there is oxidation, inflammation is not far behind; the pomegranate's powerful antioxidants are known to combat, and even prevent, chronic inflammation.

The complex and synergistic qualities of the pomegranate contribute to the fruit's unique character and rich history. Even among all the marvels of today's medicine and therapeutic nutrition, the herbal synergy within this unusual fruit has helped to highlight its modern potential.

Alzheimer's Disease

According to an animal study published in the journal *Neurobiology of Disease,* this versatile fruit may protect the nervous sys-

tem from degeneration as well. The study focused on Alzheimer's disease, the most common cause of dementia in older
adults, and a disease that has no cure. Approximately 4 million
Americans have Alzheimer's disease—roughly 1.5 percent of
the population.

> **ALZHEIMER'S DISEASE**
> A progressive disease in which nerve cells in the brain
> become damaged and brain matter shrinks, resulting
> in impaired thinking, behavior, and memory.

The study showed that pomegranate juice may offer protection against the oxidative stress that causes, and is caused by,
beta amyloid deposits. Accumulation of these harmful proteins
on neuronal cells is caused by oxidative stress, a cascade of free-
radical attacks that can kill brain cells, and contributes to the
decline of cognitive function.

Animals predisposed to Alzheimer's were given pomegranate juice. Compared with the group given a placebo, the experimental animals demonstrated superior performance in tasks
believed to require cognition. In addition, researchers deter-
mined that the amount of beta amyloid deposits in the brain
cortex of the group given pomegranate juice was 50 percent less
than in the non-supplemented group. Pomegranate juice could
be seen to actually cleanse beta amyloid deposits forming on the
neurons.

Pomegranate as a Potential Chemopreventive in Leukemia

Along with Dr. Satoru Kawaii of the Tokyo Denki University in
Saitama, Japan, Dr. Lansky investigated the effects of pomegranate extract on human leukemia cells. They wanted to deter-

mine whether pomegranate would aid in the *differentiation* of leukemia cells—the reversion of these cancerous cells back into working blood cells. Loss of differentiation of cells is one of the transformations they undergo when they become cancerous. It means they become less like other cells of the organ or system of which they are a part and stop doing their jobs in that regard. Instead, they use up energy and grow. If differentiation can be encouraged with a medicinal food such as pomegranate, this might provide a good chemopreventive alternative for leukemia as well as breast and prostate cancers.

Lansky and Kawaii tested flavonoid-rich fractions from fresh and fermented pomegranate juices, and from a water extract of peel against lines of leukemia cells. Both the fermented juice and the peel extracts strongly promoted differentiation.

Pomegranate Juice for Gastrointestinal Conditions

Pomegranate juice, with its strong astringency, can be useful for reducing swelling, and it has been used topically to treat hemorrhoids, blood vessels in the rectum that have become distended and can be painful.

ASTRINGENT
A substance that contracts the tissues or canals of the body, diminishing discharges like mucus and blood.

Some suggest that ingesting pomegranate juice can also benefit hemorrhoids, which are common during pregnancy. Tannic acids found abundantly in the rind of the pomegranate are also strongly astringent, and can help to reduce inflammatory congestion and firm up weakened tissues. They may be found in some skincare products with pomegranate ingredients.

The next time you're stricken with a bout of diarrhea, try

drinking some pomegranate juice. Its astringent qualities benefit this condition as well. Pomegranate seed extract has a long tradition of being used to destroy intestinal parasites. Orally, the juice has been used as a gargle for sore throats and mouth sores.

Common Roots of Disease Call for Common Solutions

Chronic inflammation, oxidation, and insulin resistance are proving to be common factors affecting many issues of human health. The ancient pomegranate, whose multifaceted nutritious utility was so clearly recognized and revered in the past, is now the subject of new investigations. After many centuries, pomegranate is approaching center stage as a kind of Great Red Hope.

The chapters that follow will elaborate on the journey of this celebrated yet mysterious fruit from a symbol of the spiritual, royal, and sensual to a well-elaborated medicine chest of phytochemicals for human health.

3

Women's Health

Some Biblical scholars insist that the fruit from which Eve took the first forbidden bite was not the apple, but the pomegranate. While the forbidden fruit has symbolized the source of human troubles, today the lovely pomegranate is recognized as a source of numerous benefits specific to women.

Recent research suggests that the pomegranate, rich in flavonoids, may be effective at treating and possibly preventing breast cancer. Moreover, this fruit may help with the depression and bone loss associated with menopause. Phytoestrogens from pomegranate seeds have been shown to reduce some of the symptoms of menopause through gentle, mild stimulation of estrogen receptors—hormone receptors that, following menopause, lose effectiveness.

Pomegranate Phytoestrogens

Pomegranate seeds, the white interior of the juicy arils, are 18 percent oil. Once that oil is extracted, seed cake remains. Seed cake contains bioactive plant chemicals, including lignins and polysaccharides, from which the cell walls of the seeds are built. It is the main repository of the plant's phytoestrogenic compounds. Lignans are phytoestrogenic (estrogen-like compounds found in certain plant foods) and appear to have cancer-preventive properties, particularly in women. These compounds may also reduce the risk of osteoporosis.

Phytoestrogens and Fertility

It is believed that the effects of these physiologically potent compounds on the body's hormonal systems derive from the plant's defense against being consumed by animals. Specifically, the phytoestrogens reduce the fertility of the animals that consume them. Rather than utilizing poisons against foraging

Lignans

Lignans and lignins sound alike, and in fact, they are related. Lignins are extremely strong fibers found in plants and are highly water-repellent (hydrophobic). Part of their structure includes active antioxidant elements, which also form the basis for phyto-estrogenic lignans. These are fibers as well. The lignans in food are more accurately described as lignan *precursors*. These lignan precursors are transformed by bacteria in the intestinal tract into mammalian lignans, primarily *enterodiol* and *enterolactone,* that naturally reside there. Flaxseeds are the best-known source of lignans, and pomegranate seeds may represent an alternative.

Overall, research suggests a relationship between the amount of lignan made in the body from lignan precursors and a reduced risk of breast and endometrial cancers. As weak estrogens, lignans can occupy estrogen receptors, blocking the more aggressive growth-stimulating effect of other estrogens. They can also reduce the activity of enzymes involved in estrogen metabolism, potentially reducing the production of more carcinogenic types of estrogen in the body. One Danish study found that a diet high in lignan precursors (other food sources include fruit, legumes, vegetables, and whole grains) reduced the risk of estrogen-receptor-negative animals as many plants do, the pomegranate and other phyto-estrogen-bearing species employ the tactic of altering the hormonal balance of the animals that eat them. These animals can then eat such plants in moderation, but not so fast that the animal's own potential for procreation is threatened. Other plants that employ this method include clover, flax, and soy.

Paradoxically, pomegranate is recognized worldwide for women trying to conceive, as well as for women who are pregnant. Studies show that antioxidant-rich diets are especially

breast cancer, usually considered more difficult to treat than estrogen-receptor-positive breast cancer. Another study, on Canadian women, found those who had consumed more lignan precursors in adolescence had a significantly reduced risk of breast cancer later in life. Women with higher levels of urinary enterolactone have been found to have decreased risk of endometrial and ovarian cancers, and higher urinary enterolactone was associated with higher hip-bone density in a study of Korean women.

Estrogens prescribed for female hormone replacement therapy (HRT) have pronounced bone-preserving effects, reducing the risk of osteoporosis in a population at great risk for this disease. HRT has also been found to offer substantial protection against colorectal cancer in menopausal women. Recent studies have found, however, that the typical HRT regimen—estrogens plus progestins—incurs an unacceptable increase in risk of breast cancer, heart attacks, and strokes. Research suggests that lignan precursors in the diet may serve to offer protection against osteoporosis and colorectal cancer, without the attendant risks seen from conventional HRT.

While soy foods receive the most press as phytoestrogen sources, lignan precursors are the most abundant source of dietary phytoestrogens in the typical Western diet.

crucial for women who are currently expecting or who plan to be in the future. As is common in science, the active compounds in pomegranate can produce different effects under different circumstances.

As far back as the 1960s, pomegranate seed oil was touted as having "more estrogen than any other plant source." This was long before phytoestrogen was a household word, and the compounds referred to were not the isoflavones found in clover and soybeans, but steroid hormones with the exact same structure as the human estrogens, estrone and estriol.

Estrone is a strong estrogen, but not nearly as strong as 17-beta-estradiol, which is the strongest estrogen produced by the human body. Both estrone and 17-beta-estradiol are used in conventional hormone replacement therapy (HRT), but both, unfortunately, promote growth of breast cancer cells. Indeed, HRT is the source of much controversy.

Women have been encouraged to use HRT to eliminate menopausal symptoms and prevent osteoporosis, but large research studies indicate an unacceptable increase in breast cancer risk with this therapy. Weaker plant estrogens, which are believed to be safer, non-carcinogenic alternatives, appear to be good substitutes for some women.

It's not unusual to find substances in foods that simulate the action of human sex-steroid hormones. Pomegranate, though, appears to contain versions of these hormones that are bio-identical to hormones made in the human body. Researchers even isolated testosterone from pomegranate seed oil.

The mirror image of 17-beta-estradiol is 17-alpha-estradiol. The two *isomers* are identical to one another in the same way you and your mirror image are identical. They're the same hormone, turned in opposite directions, yielding a substantial difference in physiological activity.

Both compounds are alike in that they are extremely potent

antioxidants and protectors of the brain. Both may be successful in alleviating symptoms of hot flashes, but only 17-beta-
estradiol is carcinogenic. The curious thing about these mirror-
image hormones is that while 17-beta-estradiol is the most
potent of all the steroidal estrogens produced by humans, 17-
alpha-estradiol is the mildest. Pomegranate seed is a rich source
of safe, bioactive phytoestrogens that may help women main-
tain their reproductive and menopausal health.

Pomegranate for Menopausal Symptoms

As women's hormone levels decrease during and after menopause—whether undergone naturally in their forties or fifties,
or earlier due to hysterectomy or chemotherapy—they can experience symptoms ranging from minor discomforts and incon-
veniences to more serious long-term conditions. The abrupt
loss of activity by the hormones estrogen and progesterone can
predispose a woman to many unpleasant short-term menopausal symptoms.

• Hot flashes

• Insomnia

• Mood swings

• Night sweats

Premarin and progestin, the standard HRT drugs prescribed
to women who are going through menopause, are functionally
and chemically different from the natural hormones produced
by the female body, and studies show that they are only safe for
very short-term use. The Food and Drug Administration (FDA)
recently mandated a warning for the package labels and information inserts of synthetic estrogen and progesterone products,
requiring notice of increased associated risk for breast cancer,

heart attacks, heart disease, and strokes. The warning also notes that these drugs are not approved for prevention of heart disease. Menopausal women are vulnerable to the following long-term signs of hormone deficiency:

- Anxiety

- Coronary heart disease

- Depression

- Increased cholesterol

- Irritability

- Memory loss

- Osteoporosis resulting from decreased bone density

- Thickening facial hair

- Thinning scalp hair

- Urinary incontinence

- Vaginal dryness

Foods such as pomegranate, rich in gentle, natural phyto-estrogens, may provide a solution for women wishing to avoid the risks of conventional HRT but also wanting to feel and function well for their decades beyond menopause.

With the potential risks of drug-based HRT, some women opt for an alternative approach to treating the undesirable symptoms associated with menopause. One option is to take advantage of natural forms of estrogen, such as the phytoestrogens in the pomegranate. Pomegranate probably contains a wider range of phytoestrogens than any other plant. The estrogenic richness of pomegranate encompasses not only steroidal estrogens, such as estradiols, estriol, and estrone, but also phytoestrogenic flavonoids, like luteolin, naringenin, and quercetin. Other food products with a less rich endowment of phytoestrogens include flaxseed and legumes (beans, lentils, peas, soy).

In adequate doses, phytoestrogens can stimulate biological activity comparable to endogenous (occurring naturally in the body) estrogens. Thus, a growing body of research is establishing the potential of phytoestrogens for treating or preventing menopausal symptoms. And as a result, concentrated pomegranate products, such as pomegranate seed-extract capsules and tablets, are readily available today for women who can benefit from a natural form of estrogen as part of their HRT protocol.

> ### PROGESTERONE
> A steroid hormone secreted by the ovary until menopause; counteracts growth-promoting effects of estrogen, helping to decrease risk of hormone-related cancers.

Flavonols, such as kaempferol and quercetin, both found abundantly in pomegranate, are mild phytoestrogens that also regulate many cell biochemical reactions and have profound physiological effects. The related flavone, luteolin, also found in pomegranate, has about five to six times the estrogenic activity of quercetin or kaempferol, and 58 percent of the estrogenic activity of genistein (the best known isoflavone in soybeans).

Apigenin, which binds to benzodiazepine receptors in the brain, is found in pomegranate leaves and can reduce anxiety. The effect may come from that flavone's progesterone-like activity. Progesterone is the estrogens' natural counterpart, balancing the latter hormones' growth-promoting effects and helping to relax and calm the body and mind. Pomegranate is one of the rare plant foods that contains progesterone-like compounds.

A study by researchers at Japan's Saitama Prefectural Uni-

versity employed concentrated pomegranate juice and seed
extract in an effort to improve bone health and depression in an
animal model of menopause. Ovariectomized mice—mice with
ovaries removed—were fed pomegranate juice and seed extract,
reported to contain estrone, estradiol, and estriol, as well as the
isoflavones genistein and daidzein. The loss of bone mass typical in these mice, which parallels the increasing bone loss seen
in menopausal women, was prevented.

Help for People with Breast Cancer

According to the American Cancer Society, with the exception
of non-melanoma skin cancers, breast cancer is the most common cancer among women. Women face about a one-in-eight
chance (13 percent) of developing invasive breast cancer at
some time in their lives. Those living in North America have
the highest rate of breast cancer in the world, and in 2006,
approximately 212,920 new cases of invasive breast cancer
were diagnosed among women in the United States alone.

Death rates from breast cancer have been declining, however,
most probably as a result of early detection and improved treatment. Treatments include chemotherapy, hormone therapy,
radiation, and surgery, yet many women are also including complementary therapies, such as naturopathic medicine, mind-
body medicine (psychoneuroimmunology, or PNI), and nutrition.

If the notion of using a plant or food to support cancer treatment seems far-fetched, keep in mind that some of our most
powerful chemotherapeutic agents are derived from plants. The
chemotherapy drug vincristine is found in the periwinkle plant;
Paclitaxel and Taxol are from the yew tree. Of course, these
drugs are essentially poisons, crafted by drug researchers from
plants in an effort to kill rapidly multiplying cancer cells while
doing minimal damage to healthy tissues. So far, the science of
cancer chemotherapy has been enormously challenging; these

drugs can ravage the body of the cancer patient, and sometimes the cure is as much a threat as the disease. As cancer becomes better understood, science recognizes that a better approach is to detect the disease as early as possible and then use balanced therapies with dual functions: to target the growing cancer before it can spread and become a serious threat, and to reinforce the body's natural defenses against the disease. Once again, promoting a physiological state where inflammation and oxidation are minimized seems essential.

Early detection and medical treatments for breast cancer are constantly improving, and most women survive the disease and never have a recurrence. The natural progression of breast cancer research is to design interventions that can be used to target the disease before it even really starts. Our work on developing chemopreventive agents from pomegranate is in this vein.

In 2002, Dr. Lansky directed an international group of scientists from Korea, Israel, Britain, and America in assessing the effect of subfractions of organic, fresh pomegranate—the seed oil, fermented juice, and peel extract—on the growth of human breast cancer cells. The group found that:

- Polyphenols from pomegranate juice and peel blocked estrogen synthesis in breast cancer cell cultures, inhibiting the *aromatase* enzyme by 60–80 percent.

- Fresh pomegranate juice inhibited the estrogenic activity of 17-beta-estradiol, the form of estrogen made in the body that can accelerate the growth of breast cancer cells by 55 percent.

- Fermented pomegranate-juice polyphenols showed the strongest inhibitory effects on breast cancer cell growth; fresh pomegranate juice had some cancer-inhibitory effect.

- Pomegranate seed oil significantly inhibited the proliferation of cancer cells in two different breast cancer cell lines, and stimulated *apoptosis,* the programmed death of cancerous cells.

- Polyphenols from fermented pomegranate juice inhibited the formation of a breast cancer lesion stimulated by a carcinogenic chemical called DMBA by 47 percent.

This study revealed the promise of pomegranate as a source of chemopreventive medicines that could protect women against breast cancer.

AROMATASE

A naturally occurring enzyme in the human body that transforms male hormones (androgens) into estrogens. Aromatase inhibitors are important treatments for hormone-related cancers, including those of the breast and prostate.

Pomegranate versus Angiogenesis

In a subsequent study, Dr. Lansky and co-workers from Tokyo Metropolitan Komagome Hospital in Tokyo, Japan, investigated the *anti-angiogenic* potential of pomegranate fractions. Angiogenesis describes the body's process of building new blood vessels to bring blood and nutrients to an area. In the heart, for example, an artery clogged with cholesterol-laden plaque may sprout a new vessel to bypass the clot; here, angiogenesis is salutary. But cancerous tumors can build new vessels as well, establishing their own blood and fuel supply and enabling their rapid growth. Inhibiting angiogenesis is a major route through which cancer researchers are working to eradicate cancer, or at least make it a curable disease or a disease that can be controlled.

Having demonstrated how effectively the various components of pomegranate slow the growth of breast cancer cell lines, provide positive antioxidant and anti-inflammatory effects, and favorably affect eicosanoid balance, the group collaborated with Professor Masakazu Toi, in Japan, on another study. The study found that pomegranate fractions suppressed the expression of biochemicals produced by cells as they begin the process of angiogenesis.

Finally, Dr. Lansky with Professor Rajendra-Mehta at the Department of Surgical Oncology at the University of Illinois College of Medicine used a mouse mammary organ culture to determine whether pomegranate extracts would prevent or slow the growth of breast cancer in response to exposure to the carcinogen DMBA. The mammary glands were treated for ten days with fermented pomegranate juice containing polyphenols, a highly refined extract of those polyphenols, or pomegranate seed oil. On the third day, they were exposed to DMBA. The fermented polyphenol-rich juice effected a 42 percent reduction in the number of breast cancer lesions that formed. The seed oil and the refined polyphenol extract, however, were more than twice as effective, each reducing the tumor count by 87 percent.

Overall, this research is quite promising, and will likely yield fruit—in the form of a concentrated, highly specific extract from fermented polyphenols and/or seed oil in the not-too-distant future.

Estrogens—A Danger to Women with Breast Cancer?

Women who have been diagnosed with breast cancer, or who are at elevated risk, are told to stay away from estrogens, as these hormones have growth-promoting effects on most breast cancers. These women are even told to avoid bio-identical estrogens, such as 17-beta-estradiol. Are the estrogens found in the pomegranate worthy of concern for women who have breast cancer or are at high risk for the disease? No—women probably have no need to worry about pomegranate in this regard. The

concentrations of bio-identical estrogens (in the seeds) and phytoestrogens (in the fruit and juice) are not adequate to raise
concerns about promoting the growth of breast cancer. According to published studies, unlike its 17-beta sister, 17-alpha-
estradiol does not promote cancer.

In the two-thirds of breast cancers that are estrogen-receptor
positive, the body's estrogens stimulate the proliferation of
tumor cells. Recent laboratory research has found that the phytoestrogens in pomegranate can alter the way cells respond to
the body's own estrogen. And polyphenolic substances in pomegranates have been shown to block the activity of the enzyme
aromatase, which is involved in the synthesis of estrogen. Both
laboratory findings suggest that the pomegranate may have a
place in breast cancer treatment regimens.

Scientists studied the effect of pomegranate seed extract on
breast cancer cells in a laboratory environment. They discovered that the extract reduced the activity of 17-beta-estradiol—
the estrogen of concern in breast cancer—by 50 percent.
Additionally, breast cancer cells that experienced this reduction
in estrogen stimulation died with a significantly greater frequency than normal cells.

Breast Cancer Prevention

In the face of epidemics, scientific research has often empowered
people to defend themselves—getting vaccines for flu prevention, choosing to give up smoking to reduce the risk of getting
lung cancer and other heart and lung diseases, and lowering
blood pressure to ward off strokes. Although women have felt
powerless to prevent breast cancer in the past, extensive research
in recent decades has armed them with important information
and useful tools for protection. Through these widespread studies, nutrition is emerging as a key component of preventing
breast cancer. Nutrition might even be the *most* powerful meas-

ure the majority of women can take against breast cancer. (Genetic predisposition is another question but nutritional intervention can still play an important role.) Researchers at the Simone Protective Cancer Institute of New Jersey point out that 90 percent of all cancers could be traced back to smoking and dietary, or nutritional, factors. Diets rich in nutritional chemopreventive substances—nutrients and phytochemicals that delay, forestall, or even reverse the growth cycle of cancerous cells—are an important avenue to cancer prevention.

So, while age and family history are associated with an increased risk of breast cancer, much research suggests that women are not helpless in the face of this disease. They can take charge through nutritional programs designed to prevent the disease from ever occurring.

PHYTOCHEMICAL
A large, general class of compounds that includes vitamins, minerals, and other naturally occurring nutrients and non-nutritive substances in plants.

Some of the latest research concerning breast cancer prevention underscores the importance of diets rich in various superfoods and nutrients. The recommendations include olive oil, broccoli, cabbage, cauliflower, and other cruciferous vegetables (for their indole-3-carbinol), carrots (for their carotenoids), fish oil (for its docosahexaenoic acid, or DHA, an omega-3 polyunsaturated fatty acid), green tea (for its polyphenols and catechins), foods high in folic acid and the B vitamins, fruits and vegetables containing beta-carotene and glucaric acid, and foods low in saturated fats. One of the newer foods to hit this list of chemopreventive substances is the pomegranate, a rich source of ellagic acid and related compounds.

> **CHEMOPREVENTION**
> The use of chemical agents, drugs, or food nutrients
> to prevent disease.

Ellagic Acid for Cancer Chemoprevention

While research suggests that ellagic acid has the ability to prevent, inhibit, reduce the numbers of, and even destroy cancer cells, research has demonstrated that it is the complex ellagic-acid containing tannins that actually work far better than ellagic acid alone. Ellagic acid appears to be a good protector due to its ability to induce cellular detoxification enzymes, including the flavoprotein NAD(P)H:quinine reductase (QR). These enzymes have been shown to increase the detoxification of carcinogens and reduce carcinogen-induced mutations and tumors. A University of Kentucky Graduate Center for Toxicology study shows that ellagic acid inhibits the earliest chemical reactions that can lead to the development of breast cancer.

In another study, the Hollings Cancer Center at the Medical University of South Carolina found that ellagic acid was able to prevent cancer even in those with a genetic predisposition to the disease. Additionally, the studies found that ellagic acid slows the growth of abnormal colon cells, promotes the natural death (apoptosis) of prostate cancer cells, and prevents the development of cells infected with human papilloma virus (HPV), which is linked to cervical cancer. Ellagic acid's apoptotic properties have also been found to slow or stop the growth of breast, esophageal, lung, and skin cancers.

Reducing the Risk of Infant Brain Injury

Decreased oxygen and blood flow to an infant's brain is linked to premature birth and other irregularities of pregnancy, including seizures and cerebral palsy. Approximately two out of every 1,000 full-term births, and a relatively high percentage of babies born before thirty-four weeks of gestation, develop hypoxia-ischemia that leads to brain injury.

A recent study in mice suggests that expectant women at risk for a premature birth can drink pomegranate juice during pregnancy to help reduce the risk of ischemia and brain injuries in their babies.

> **ISCHEMIA**
> Blood flow and oxygen to cells and organs that is insufficient to maintain their normal function.

In a 2005 report from the Washington University School of Medicine in St. Louis, researchers fed pregnant mice with pomegranate concentrate and water, while a control group of pregnant mice drank other fluids. They then briefly lowered the levels of brain blood and oxygen in the newborn mice. The group of mice whose mothers consumed pomegranate juice lost 60 percent less brain tissue than the latter group, and these results strongly suggest that antioxidant polyphenols in pomegranate have a protective role against hypoxic brain damage.

Investigators were able to conclude from the study that an enzyme, capsase-3, was 84 percent less active in mice whose mothers drank pomegranate juice. Capsase-3 is a part of the self-destruction process in oxygen-starved brain cells—the kind of apoptosis (cell death) you don't want. When you are trying to slow or stop cancer growth, apoptosis is desirable.

Antioxidant polyphenols, found abundantly in pomegranate, have been intensely studied for their neuroprotective effects. Medical experts say that treating hypoxic ischemic brain injury is quite difficult. However, preventing those diseases in the first place with nutrition—specifically, antioxidant compounds from pomegranate—is a solution more likely to succeed. Because of all the technologies at our disposal, knowing who is at risk for premature birth is easier today.

Women must concern themselves with menopausal, menstrual, and related health issues. Pomegranate can support women's health throughout their lives—and it can do so with taste!

4

Men's Health

We've established that the pomegranate has much to offer women and, as so often turns out, what's good for the goose is sauce for the gander. Men can also turn to the pomegranate for help with gender-specific conditions.

Awareness of male prostate health is at an all-time high, thanks to numerous high-profile males speaking openly about their prostate conditions. Erectile dysfunction, once a private and discreet discussion between a man and his doctor, has now become a high-profile item on the American advertising agenda, due in no small part to a new fascination with pharmaceuticals touted for countering this condition. Yet, the appeal of such items has been perennial; aphrodisiacs and performance enhancers being both ancient and universal.

Nowadays, studies show that pomegranate juice can slow the progression of prostate cancer, and its potent, anti-inflammatory antioxidants aid in preventing or relieving symptoms of an enlarged prostate. Furthermore, the fruit also has been shown to improve penile blood flow and erectile response.

Prostate Cancer

According to the American Cancer Society, after skin cancer, prostate cancer is the second most common type of cancer in American men. It is the third leading cause of cancer death in men, after lung and colorectal cancers. One out of six men will get prostate cancer during his lifetime, yet only one in thirty-four will die of the disease. Usually, a man will die of old age or another condition first since prostate cancer is generally slow growing. The slowness of growth roughly correlates to the age of the patient at the onset of the disease.

As with other cancers, prostate cancer is being detected earlier today thanks to diagnostic improvements, and the death rate for this cancer is falling as well. Some prostate cancers are small and do not grow rapidly, so aggressive treatment is not usually required. Surgical techniques have come a long way since the time when treatment for prostate cancer was almost always the complete removal of the prostate gland—a surgery that, in those times, often caused impotence and/or incontinence. Up-to-date laser procedures, cryotherapy, and other high-tech surgeries now enable physicians to more precisely target diseased tissues and remove or kill them without harming the nerves that bring sensation and muscle control to the bladder and erectile tissues.

The most common tests for prostate cancer include checking the amount of prostate-specific antigen (PSA) in the blood and performing a digital rectal exam (DRE). Men are advised to begin having yearly PSA and DRE tests starting at age fifty (African-American men and men with a family history of prostate cancer by age forty-five).

It is not yet known what causes prostate cancer, but the American Cancer Society suggests that certain risk factors are linked to the disease including age, family history, nationality, race, diet, and exercise. Men with diets high in red meat or high-fat dairy products seem to show a higher incidence. Significantly, these same men also frequently eat fewer fruits and vegetables. Though doctors aren't certain which of these factors causes the risk to go up, they recommend eating at least five servings of vegetables and fruits daily, and consuming less red meat and fewer high-fat dairy products.

PROSTATE-SPECIFIC ANTIGEN
A protein produced in the prostate gland, and shown to be elevated in men with prostate cancer and enlarged prostates.

Certain dietary extracts have been found to reduce the growth of prostate cancer cells. Chemopreventive dietary intervention may prove helpful in reducing and stabilizing prostate tumors. Pomegranate is one of the more promising candidates for prostate cancer chemoprevention.

Though today's prostate cancer treatments are known to cure two-thirds of men with the disease, following treatment, one-third of these men show rising levels of their PSA. Of that one-third, 34 percent progress to fatal prostate cancer within fifteen years. The faster PSA levels rise following treatment, the sooner a man's prostate cancer is likely to return. Many men with prostate cancer who face rising PSA levels opt for drugs that block testosterone, but this treatment can have serious side effects, including bone loss, sexual dysfunction, and depression.

Several intriguing studies have been published on the use of pomegranate for prostate cancer prevention and treatment. One such study, performed at the University of Wisconsin and published in the *Proceedings of the National Academy of Sciences* in 2005, describes an experiment where highly aggressive prostate cancer cells were treated with a pomegranate fruit extract. There was a **dose-dependent** inhibition of cancer-cell growth and viability, and apoptosis was induced.

In this study, not only were pro-apoptotic changes seen, but *anti*-apoptotic aspects of the cells were down-regulated—in other words, the pomegranate treatment appeared to enhance apoptosis in more than one way. These same investigators then administered the pomegranate extract to mice implanted with prostate tumors. There was a significant inhibition in tumor growth and a reduction in PSA levels.

> **DOSE-DEPENDENT**
> A term used in medical research to describe increasing responsiveness of the treated entity to increasing doses of the treatment.

In collaboration with scientists in Germany, Israel, the Netherlands, Britain, and America, Dr. Lansky completed a multi-center study of the effects of pomegranate seed oil, fermented juice polyphenols, and polyphenols from pomegranate rind on prostate cancer cell growth, proliferation, migration, and apoptosis. The group found these parts of the pomegranate to acutely inhibit the proliferation (the growth of more cancerous cells) of two human prostate cancer cell lines. Supercritical carbon dioxide–extracted pomegranate seed oil extract was found to potently inhibit the growth of prostate cancer cells grafted to mice. The overall results of this study demonstrated an extremely promising role for pomegranate derivatives against prostate cancer in men.

A landmark clinical study was recently completed at UCLA's David Geffen School of Medicine. Men who had undergone surgery or radiation therapy for prostate cancer were given eight ounces of pomegranate juice daily and monitored for rising PSA. At the study's outset, all the subjects had already been found to have rising PSA levels, indicating a possible recurrence of disease.

Men who supplemented with pomegranate juice experienced a delayed rise in their PSA following prostate cancer treatment.

In these men, the mean PSA doubling time went from fifteen months to an astounding fifty-four months. In addition, patient serum added to a prostate cancer cell line in a test tube caused a 12 percent drop in cell proliferation and a 17 percent increase in apoptosis, suggesting the person's body was better equipped to resist the growth of cancer. Significant decreases in the oxidative state and in LDL oxidation were also seen in this study. Compared to a control group who got no juice, the PSA-escalation time was nearly four times slower in the men who consumed the juice.

> **SUPERCRITICAL EXTRACTION**
> A method of extracting oils or other active constituents from plants using either carbon dioxide or water at the supercritical point, the interphase between the gaseous and liquid phase. The procedure leaves the extracted product free of toxic solvent residues.

More than one-third of the men in the pomegranate group showed a decrease in PSA levels, and in four of the forty-six men who ingested the juice, PSA levels dropped by half. The men in the study who continued drinking pomegranate juice daily for more than three years kept their PSA levels steady. Conclusion? Drinking pomegranate juice daily can suppress prostate cancer growth in men threatened by the recurrence of a tumor.

The UCLA research team reported that "pomegranate juice is a very non-toxic treatment that, if it really did have that effect of doubling time, could prevent many people from going on to metastatic disease and . . . dying of prostate cancer." They postulated that ingredients in pomegranate juice may be involved in prostate cancer prevention, but could not say exactly how the juice exerted its dramatic effect.

A 2005 study performed at the University of Wisconsin and published in the *Proceedings of the National Academy of Sciences* showed similar results. The study evaluated the anti-proliferative and pro-apoptotic properties of pomegranate-fruit extract in mouse skin, using human prostate cancer cells. The results further underscored the potential preventive and therapeutic effects of pomegranate on prostate cancer. The pomegranate-fruit extract inhibited the cell growth and cell viability of highly aggressive human prostate cancer cells. Researchers concluded that pomegranate juice may have cancer-chemotherapeutic as well as cancer-chemopreventive effects against prostate cancer in humans.

APOPTOSIS
A form of cell self-destruction, also known
as programmed cell death.

At this writing, a team led by Aaron Katz, M.D., director of the New York Presbyterian Hospital/Columbia Holistic Urology Center is investigating the effects of an extract of pomegranate and lycopene on the progression of prostate cancer. The possibility that the efficacy of pomegranate in this and other conditions might be enhanced by other medicinal foods, such as the tomato, is implied in this particular investigation.

Some evidence points to estrogens as initiators or accelerators of prostate cancer growth because, as they age, men tend to aromatize (transform with the help of the enzyme aromatase) more of their testosterone into growth-promoting estrogens. With aging, men's aromatase activity tends to rise, causing an increase in estrogenic stimulation of the prostate gland. Thus, the gentle phytoestrogenic effects of pomegranate and its inhibitory effects on the enzyme aromatase could help protect against prostate cancer.

Enlarged Prostate

Though most men will be fortunate enough to dodge prostate cancer, many more will eventually develop an enlarged prostate, known as benign prostatic hyperplasia (BPH).

The prostate is a gland approximately the shape and size of a walnut. It surrounds the urethra, the tube through which urine travels from the bladder to exit the body. During puberty, when testosterone levels rise, the prostate grows rapidly, doubling in size by age twenty. For the next two decades, the growth slows down. According to the American Urological Association, the prostate doesn't usually cause problems for many years, with less than 10 percent of thirty-year-old men having an enlarged prostate. By age forty, the prostate typically goes through a second growth spurt. By the age of sixty, over half of men have a clinically enlarged prostate. By age eighty-five, 90 percent of men are affected. The enlargement does not affect urine flow in every case; sometimes, the gland grows in size without pressing inward on the urethra. In others, though, even a slight amount of prostatic growth can precipitate urinary troubles.

BPH is a non-cancerous enlargement of the prostate that puts pressure on the urethra, blocking urine flow. As blockage increases, the bladder muscle has to push harder to get its job done. This dynamic can lead to irritability or oversensitivity of the bladder. Symptoms include a weak or slow urinary flow, a feeling of incomplete bladder emptying, urinary frequency or urgency, or frequent urination during the nighttime.

> **BENIGN PROSTATIC HYPERPLASIA**
> Also known as BPH or enlarged prostate; a non-cancerous enlargement of the prostate gland, common in middle-aged and older men.

When the bladder doesn't completely empty, men can be at risk for developing urinary tract infections. In rare cases, bladder or kidney damage, bladder stones, blood in the urine, inability to urinate, and incontinence can develop from BPH. Many treatments exist for BPH, including medications, minimally invasive procedures, and surgery, but side effects are common and all have potential complications.

Enter the pomegranate, specifically its rich store of anti-inflammatory phytochemicals. A recent Mayo Clinic study noted that anti-inflammatory drugs may prevent enlarged prostate symptoms. The eighteen-year study of more than 2,400 men proved that men who took a daily dose of over-the-counter anti-inflammatory drugs showed 50 percent or less risk of developing an enlarged prostate than the control group. Dosage didn't seem to matter, as researchers said the same apparent protective effects of the anti-inflammatory drugs were seen at both low and high doses. The researchers also cautioned men against taking the drugs if they weren't already prescribed for another condition, since non-steroidal anti-inflammatory drugs (NSAIDs) can cause bleeding gastric ulcers.

Pomegranate juice, peel, and seed oil, on the other hand, are all known to possess natural anti-inflammatory compounds that can combat chronic inflammation. For example, pomegranate seed oil is one of only about six plant sources known to contain conjugated fatty acids, including punicic acid. These conjugated fatty acids inhibit eicosanoid metabolism in the synthesis of prostaglandins from arachidonic acid, an omega-6 fatty acid—the same mechanism by which NSAIDs control inflammation.

Recall, too, that pomegranates contain anthocyanins, a subclass of polyphenols that are important antioxidants. When consumed, they protect tissues from the oxidative damage caused by free radicals, thereby helping to break the downward spiral of inflammation and oxidation, which, not surprisingly, has been implicated in BPH.

Erectile Dysfunction

As men age, they face a greater potential for experiencing erectile dysfunction (ED). In a 2003 Harvard School of Public Health survey involving 31,742 men between the ages of fifty-three and ninety, 33 percent reported experiencing ED in the previous three months. Yet, fewer than 2 percent reported experiencing such difficulties before age forty. Thus, from age fifty on up, the percentage of men reporting ED increased dramatically.

> **ERECTILE DYSFUNCTION**
> Also known as impotence or ED; the inability of men to obtain and sustain an erection adequate for intercourse.

Prescription drugs such as Cialis, Levitra, and Viagra are the most commonly prescribed treatments. Other available options include implants, vacuum devices, and vascular surgery; some men have benefited from psychotherapy. Before prescribing a pill or surgery, the modern physician might recommend pomegranate juice for his or her ED patients.

A 2005 study published in the *Journal of Urology* examined the effects of long-term consumption of antioxidant beverages, including blueberry juice, cranberry juice, green tea, orange juice, pomegranate juice, and red wine, on ED in rabbits. The results suggest that free radicals are a contributing factor in ED in rabbits, and the same may indeed prove so in humans.

Pomegranate juice showed the greatest capacity of all the preparations tested to decrease low-density lipoprotein (LDL) oxidation, and had the greatest inhibitory effect on oxidative stress in macrophages (immune cells). The juice increased penile blood flow, improved erectile response and smooth-muscle relaxation, and prevented erectile-tissue fibrosis (oxidative tissue damage that can lead to permanent erectile problems) in the group with ED.

Many of the wonderful benefits that the pomegranate offers, such as help for cardiovascular disease, aging, and osteoarthritis, apply to both sexes. The support it lends to reproductive health is another benefit common to both sexes. Eating pomegranates and drinking its juice is the simplest way to reap these benefits. Using supplements that contain extracts of the whole fruit, including concentrated pomegranate seed oil rich in conjugated fatty acids, may provide a viable alternative.

5

Your Heart Will Love Pomegranates

". . . Pomegranate . . . if cut deep down the middle, shows
a heart within blood-tinctured, of a veined humanity."
—ELIZABETH BARRETT BROWNING, *LADY GERALDINE'S COURTSHIP*

To the ancient Chinese alchemists, the pomegranate's blood-red color was a sign of immortality. The Doctrine of Signatures suggests that the pomegranate's color, shape, and size are a hint from Mother Nature that this food is good for the heart.

Studies show that just two ounces of pomegranate juice daily can help preserve the health of the cardiovascular system, which includes the heart itself and the many arteries that feed its muscular walls. Considering the prevalence of heart disease in America, this is good news. Cardiovascular disease (CVD) is the leading cause of death in both men and women in the United States and most of the world.

CVD is not a single disease, but rather a group of interrelated conditions that affect the heart, blood vessels, and blood cells. A heart attack or occlusive stroke (where a clot or other blockage cuts off blood supply to a part of the brain) is the culmination of many years of small shifts in the health of the cardiovascular system's many parts. Early intervention in the development of cardiovascular disease with dietary changes that have been conclusively shown to preserve cardiovascular health is part of a solid strategy for prevention.

According to the American Heart Association, there are currently more than 71 million American adults with at least one
form of cardiovascular disease. However, even once the disease
has taken hold, the process that creates arterial plaques that
cause heart attacks or strokes is often reversible with aggressive
dietary and lifestyle interventions. This is a disease that is
highly responsive to nutritional support.

Pomegranate fills the bill here in several ways. The pomegranate seems to stimulate the production of nitric oxide, a
chemical that keeps arteries open and blood flowing. The juice
also appears to inhibit atherosclerosis—the development of
plaques in the coronary arteries. In fact, recent studies show
that pomegranate can decrease the oxidation that causes the
bad (low-density lipoprotein, or LDL) cholesterol to adhere to
artery walls. Other research suggests that pomegranate juice
may help reduce blood pressure.

Inhibiting Atherosclerosis

Atherosclerosis is a disease of the arteries affecting an estimated 4.6 million (1.7 percent) Americans. It primarily affects
the coronary arteries, those large vessels responsible for delivering oxygen and blood to the muscular wall of the heart. This
progressive disease develops when the blood vessel wall is
injured, beginning an inflammatory and oxidative cycle, and
promoting a buildup of fat and plaque deposits just beneath the
arterial linings. These plaques can eventually cause a nar-
rowing or complete blockage of the coronary arteries. When
atherosclerosis restricts blood flow, any number of serious
conditions can result, including heart pains (angina), irregular
heartbeats (arrhythmias), heart attacks, strokes, transient
ischemic attacks (TIAs, where the carotid artery is clogged,
causing temporary reduction of blood flow to the brain), or
erectile dysfunction.

High blood pressure, a common problem in aging individuals, is another factor that initiates and accelerates the progression of coronary artery disease. Individuals with metabolic syndrome, including blood-glucose imbalances, diabetes, insulin resistance, and obesity are at a dramatically increased risk of heart disease. Pomegranate's heart benefits described in this chapter build on those from Chapter 2.

Recent studies show that drinking pomegranate juice regularly can reverse the progression of atherosclerosis—both in its early and late stages. A more in-depth look at the process of atherosclerosis will explain how this happens.

Atherosclerosis in a Nutshell

Traditionally, the belief has been that atherosclerosis begins when LDL cholesterol binds to constituents in the artery walls, causing lipids to accumulate in the arteries as plaque. However, recent investigations have pointed more strongly to a role for micro-injuries to the blood vessel walls—possibly caused by LDL that has already been oxidized by free radicals—which then set the stage for the accumulation of lipids and other substances as inflammation sets in.

Either way, through oxidative reactions to free radicals, the trapped LDL becomes susceptible to changes in its lipid structures. These modifications initiate the activity of leukocytes, or white blood cells. The leukocytes transform into macrophages—literally, "large eaters"—and seek out the oxidized LDL. The macrophages eventually consume enough oxidized LDL to become overloaded with cholesterol, transforming themselves into "foam cells" (lipid-laden macrophages). Some foam cells leave the inner lining of the arteries, taking the cholesterol back into the circulation with them, but when more lipids enter the artery wall than leave via the macrophages or other vehicles, atherosclerosis occurs.

PLAQUE
An area where fatty material and inflammation create a
bulge along the inner lining of an arterial wall.

Pomegranate and Atherosclerosis

Numerous studies demonstrate that pomegranate slows the progression of atherosclerosis at several points along the process.
Researchers at a California university assessed pomegranate's
effect on people with ischemic coronary heart disease (CHD).

ISCHEMIA
Ischemia is where lack of oxygen damages or destroys body
tissues. This is the cause of angina pain, as well as the
damage done by heart attacks and strokes.

The study, published in the *Journal of Cardiology,* showed
that pomegranate juice seems to improve blood flow to the
heart. Participants who had CHD and myocardial (heart)
ischemia drank eight ounces of pomegranate juice daily for
three months. Blood flow to their hearts improved by about 17
percent. The researchers concluded that "daily consumption of
pomegranate juice may improve stress-induced myocardial
ischemia in patients who have CHD," and that it may in fact
help prevent CHD in people who do not already have it. Research is currently underway to investigate this latter possibility.

Another study, published in *Clinical Nutrition* in 2004,
found cardiovascular benefits in people with heart disease who
drank eight ounces of pomegranate juice daily for one year.
They experienced a 59 percent decrease in LDL susceptibility
to oxidation, up to a 30 percent decrease in arterial-wall thickness in the carotid artery (the artery in the neck that, when

occluded, causes TIAs), a 130 percent improvement in total serum antioxidant status, and even a 21 percent decrease in systolic blood pressure. Those who continued the daily dosage for two additional years maintained the positive cardiovascular effects. So, it's obvious that pomegranate juice is a supremely heart-healthy beverage.

Antioxidant Protection Reduces LDL Stickiness

An important factor in the pomegranate's ability to combat atherosclerosis is its concentration of antioxidants, one of the highest found in any juice. The antioxidant polyphenols help to reduce LDL oxidation, which reduces the affinity of LDL for arterial walls.

In several human clinical trials, pomegranate juice has effectively reduced LDL oxidation, macrophage-oxidative status, and foam cell formation, all contributors to the development of atherosclerosis. Tannins seem to be the primary components responsible for the reduction of these oxidative states, along with other polyphenols such as anthocyanins.

Heart Health—Of Mice and Men

Two studies by the Lipid Research Laboratory in Haifa, Israel— a nation with cardiovascular disease issues similar in urgency to those of the United States—shed further light on the heart-protective potential of the pomegranate. Both studies involved a special breed of mouse, bred to develop atherosclerosis: the rodent counterpart of the human couch potato with metabolic syndrome.

In the first investigation, both mice and humans were studied. The purpose was to assess the antioxidant effects of pomegranate juice in the diet against oxidation of cholesterol (LDL and HDL) over a period of two weeks (in humans) and fourteen weeks (in mice). Significant antioxidant effects were seen in the human subjects; in the mice, LDL oxidation by macrophages (which also have inflammatory effects) was reduced by up to *90 percent*. Macrophages took up 20 percent less oxidized cholesterol, which suggests that the juice intervention would slow the accumulation of foam cells along arterial walls. Atherosclerotic lesions in these mice were shrunk by 44 percent over those of control mice fed water instead of juice. This is a very potent anti-atherogenic intervention.

The second study investigated the effect of treatment of mice with severe atherosclerosis using a tannin fraction isolated from pomegranate juice. Aged mice (four years old) were given either pomegranate juice or water, the aged mice compared with young (four-month-old) mice over the course of the two-month experiment. Not surprisingly, the tannin fraction of pomegranate juice improved every parameter of cardiovascular health in the aged, plaque-ridden mice, and the size of the atherosclerotic lesions decreased by 17 percent in those that got juice. LDL oxidation was also reduced, and the progression of atherosclerosis was significantly slowed.

Enhances Activity of Lipid-Eating Enzyme

Another mechanism of the pomegranate in fighting atherosclerosis is its apparent ability to increase the activity of an important enzyme known as paraoxonase. This enzyme has been shown to destroy oxidized lipids found in LDL, preventing the formation of macrophages and foam cells. Studies show a significant elevation of paraoxonase activity in people who have recently consumed pomegranate juice.

Research also suggests that pomegranate may inhibit cholesterol metabolism in macrophages and slow their progression to foam cells. The result is faster transport of cholesterol out of atherosclerotic lesions, and possibly a slowing in the growth of those lesions.

Reducing Inflammation

The role of inflammation in the atherosclerotic process is well-established. In fact, a marker of generalized inflammation called C-reactive protein (CRP) has been as good a predictor of heart disease risk as blood cholesterol counts. Drugs with established value for the prevention of heart disease, including the statins used to lower cholesterol, usually have some anti-inflammatory effect.

In a 2002 review article in *Circulation,* authors Peter Libby, Paul Ridker, and Attilio Maseri state that "[r]ecent advances in basic science have established a fundamental role for inflammation in mediating all stages of this disease from initiation through progression and, ultimately, the thrombotic complications of atherosclerosis." Where inflammation is involved, the anti-inflammatory phytochemicals of pomegranate can play a role in prevention or healing.

The research has yet to show exactly how this might work with regard to heart health, but the profound effects of regular pomegranate juice consumption on the progression of cardiovascular disease is likely to be due, at least in part, to the anti-inflammatory benefits packed into this colorful fruit.

Pomegranate Seed Oil Rich in Cholesterol Blocking Sterols

Another exciting discovery is that pomegranate seed oil is also rich in sterols. Sterols, often called phytosterols because they are found in plants, have cholesterol-lowering effects, and have been found to bolster immunity in animals and humans.

Sterols are found in the cells and cell membranes of plants. Many occur in nature—250 sterols have been discovered so far—but the best known and most thoroughly studied are *beta-sitosterol, campesterol,* and *sigmasterol.* As far back as the 1950s, science found that such sterols could block the absorption of another sterol, cholesterol, in the intestine. In fact, cholesterol is also a sterol that is essential for life—an important component of our cell membranes. But in excess, cholesterol can be dangerous. For simplicity, "sterol" in the ensuing discussion refers to sterols other than cholesterol.

The reason for this blocking effect is that sterols and cholesterol are derivative from a common essential molecular structure. They would each be absorbed through the wall of the small intestine into the bloodstream via the same minuscule passageways. However, the difference between the two is significant enough to cause one (sterols) to be absorbed in only a tenth the amount as the other (cholesterol). Sterols effectively occupy those passageways without being absorbed, and this causes some of the cholesterol to pass through unabsorbed and be eliminated from the body.

Sterols are, at this writing, a popular addition to margarines designed to help lower cholesterol. One such margarine has been found to lower LDL cholesterol by up to 24 percent in some subjects in only four weeks. Eating pomegranate arils (including the seeds) or taking concentrated pomegranate supplements that include seed oil may provide alternative means of adding these beneficial sterols to the diet.

Reducing Hypertension

Hypertension—or high blood pressure—affects an estimated 50 million Americans. High blood pressure increases the risk of heart disease, kidney disease, peripheral vascular disease, and strokes. While dietary factors are strongly implicated in hypertension, a hereditary component seems to come into play as well. Hypertension is highly dangerous, dramatically increasing blood vessel damage and the risk for heart attacks and strokes. Recent research suggests that pomegranate may reduce blood pressure.

In an Israeli study, subjects who consumed pomegranate juice for one year saw their systolic blood pressure (the top number in the blood pressure reading representing heart contraction) fall by an average of 21 percent. In another study at the same institution, researchers gave hypertensive people pomegranate juice for two weeks. In that brief period, systolic blood pressure was reduced 5 percent.

Pomegranate juice also inhibited the activity of the angiotensin-converting enzyme (ACE), involved in raising blood pressure, by 36 percent. Inhibition of ACE is known to lead to fewer heart attacks in people with heart disease, while also helping to fight atherosclerosis. Researchers concluded that the ability of pomegranate juice to protect against cardiovascular diseases could be related to its capacity to reduce oxidative stress and ACE activity.

Blood Circulation Enhancement

Research shows that pomegranate stimulates the production of nitric oxide, a chemical with a powerful vasodilatory (blood vessel–opening) effect. In fact, the nitrate drugs taken to open tightened coronary arteries during angina attacks are a pharmaceutical form of this same chemical. Drugs used to treat erectile dysfunction operate through enhanced nitric oxide action in the blood vessels of the penis.

Nitric oxide (NO) keeps arteries open and blood flowing. The antioxidant activity of pomegranate polyphenols is reported to boost the activity of nitric-oxide synthase, an enzyme that facilitates production of NO by as much as 50 percent. This has the effect of lowering high blood pressure, improving arterial health, and increasing blood vessel dilation (opening) and blood flow to all organs.

While contemporary surgical procedures and drug therapies enable more people with heart disease to survive far longer than they ever have before, this is still a disease better prevented than treated. So far, studies find that drinking pomegranate juice can powerfully support the health of your heart and blood vessels through multiple mechanisms—another example of the power of the right foods to delay the progression of some of the most frightening, deadly, and costly diseases known to humankind.

6

The Pomegranate Diet

ver one billion adults across the globe are overweight. Some 300 million of those adults are obese. Both overweight and obesity are concerns that go far beyond any issue of fashion or beauty, as both increase the risk of certain cancers, heart disease, metabolic syndrome, strokes, and type 2 diabetes.

Before delving into the uses of pomegranate in the quest for slimming, it might be helpful to clarify the definitions of *overweight* and *obesity*. A measurement called the *Body Mass Index* (BMI) is most commonly used to determine whether a person is incurring increased health risk due to his or her weight. To figure out your BMI, divide your weight in pounds by your height in inches squared, then multiply by 703:

$$BMI = \frac{Weight\ in\ Pounds}{Height\ in\ Inches^2} \times 703$$

Let's say you weigh 160 pounds and you're 58 inches tall. First, multiply 58 times 58 to get 3,364. Then, divide 160 by 3,364 to get 0.0476, and then multiply that number by 703 to get 33.5. That number is your BMI.

If your BMI is 18.5 or less, consider yourself underweight; if it is between 18.5 and 24.9, your weight is well within normal, healthy ranges. At a BMI between 25 and 29.9, you are considered overweight; 30 to 39.9, obese; 40 or greater, extremely obese.

Beyond a BMI of 25, your body begins to undergo changes that predispose you to disease and premature aging—and these processes are linked to overweight and obesity by those important common denominators, inflammation and oxidation.

How Excess Body Fat Enhances Inflammation and Oxidation

When you put on pounds, you are storing away extra food energy in your fat cells, also known as *adipocytes*. These adipocytes were once thought of as inert storage depots for energy. Fat tissue—made up of fat cells—are, in actuality, endocrine organs that make bioactive substances such as the hormones leptin and adiponectin, as well as cytokines, biochemicals that promote the vicious cycle of inflammation and oxidation.

When adipocytes are packed full and stretched with stored fat, these cells recruit macrophages, immune mediators of inflammation. This sets off a cascade of biochemical events that is believed to cause insulin resistance and sets the stage for metabolic syndrome.

It follows that losing weight is about much more than looking good—it is about reining in a physiological process that can put ever-increasing distance between you and a state of solid good health. It follows that any food, supplement, or medicine that helps reduce the impact of inflammation and free-radical overload on the body's systems will reduce the negative impact of overweight and obesity. Pomegranate can do this, and it appears that it may also have direct slimming effects as well.

Pomegranate for Slimming?

The most important steps you can take to reduce weight are to substitute more whole, unprocessed vegetables and fruits for refined starches, sugars, and junk food and to exercise! Even walking can be a big help if done daily. Instead of reaching for a greasy fast-food cheeseburger, choose a green salad with some lean protein. Instead of snacking on chips or pretzels, reach for apples or celery sticks. Instead of rich desserts as a matter of course, make nutrient-dense fresh fruit—pomegranate—your new habit. Instead of a large cola, sip a pomegranate juice cocktail made with sparkling water. These kinds of changes may seem small, but they can shave calories from your daily diet, and this can add up to losses of ten pounds or more a year. These losses are sustainable, unlike fad diets.

While it is not a magic cure for obesity, pomegranate consumption may be helpful in controlling weight. Pomegranate contains numerous compounds that are helpful for slimming whether you're looking to shed a few pounds around the middle or contending with obesity. Exercise and a healthy diet that includes pomegranate can assist in a return from the precipice that is metabolic syndrome.

As you now know, metabolic syndrome includes a group of health problems, such as elevated blood pressure, elevated blood sugar, excessive fat around the waist, high triglycerides, and low high-density lipoprotein (HDL) cholesterol, known as the good cholesterol. Together, this group of health problems can elevate your risk of diabetes, heart attacks, and strokes.

The syndrome seems to be increasing in prevalence. Approximately 10 percent of young adults and 44 percent of those over sixty years of age show symptoms of metabolic syndrome. The syndrome is often caused by an unhealthy lifestyle—eating an excess of high-calorie foods, gaining weight, particularly around the midsection, and a lack of physical activity. Metabolic syndrome is also known as insulin resistance syndrome, dysmetabolic syndrome, and syndrome X. Additionally, metabolic syndrome is known as pre-diabetes, since the former, if left untended, often evolves into the latter.

Insulin Resistance

Insulin resistance occurs when body cells don't fully respond to the action of insulin. Insulin is a protein-hormone produced by the Islets of Langerhans in the pancreas. Although the main function of the pancreas is to secrete enzymes to digest proteins, the Islets of Langerhans cells within the pancreas secrete insulin, a compound which carefully regulates blood-sugar uptake, and consequently, many physiological functions.

In a normally functioning pancreas, insulin is constantly released into the bloodstream in small amounts. When the glucose (simple carbohydrate) in your blood rises after a meal, the Islet cells release insulin to move more glucose into the cells. This results in your blood glucose level dropping. When your blood glucose drops to a certain point, your body signals you to eat. When you eat or drink, the glucose in your food is absorbed through the wall of the small intestine into circulation. The Islets detect another surge in blood sugar and more insulin is kicked into your bloodstream.

Insulin is important for growth and in the regulation of many states of health and disease. If the process of insulin uptake by the cells is impaired, the cells enter the state known as insulin resistance. Insulin resistance typically develops in people who are overweight and don't get enough exercise. Many of these individuals also have high blood pressure and high cholesterol. Insulin resistance dramatically raises the risk of heart disease and strokes, especially if other risk factors such as high cholesterol and smoking are present.

Diabetes

Insulin resistance is an important factor in sugar diabetes—known by the medical profession as diabetes mellitus. Approximately 20 million Americans have diabetes and almost one-third are not aware of it. Another 41 million Americans have pre-diabetes and have symptoms that could lead to diabetes mellitis. As yet, there is no cure.

Healthy people produce sufficient amounts of insulin to stimulate successful glucose uptake by the cells and thus eliminate excess sugar in the blood. For those with diabetes, however, this process of insulin production and resulting sugar uptake is inefficient or nonexistent. The most common form of diabetes is type 2, which is generally diet-related. Type 1 diabetes affects mostly children and is generally *not* diet-related but believed to be caused by pancreatic autoimmunity. Early in type 2 onset, blood sugars and insulin production are high. But, it's like shouting in a noisy room. The insulin isn't heard by the cells, and the cells don't do its bidding by letting glucose in. Both high blood sugars and high insulin levels are damaging to arterial walls, predisposing individuals to atherosclerosis (coronary artery disease). The inner layers of the arterial walls become thick and irregular due to injury, inflammation, and the resulting deposits of fat, cholesterol, and other substances. Eventually, insulin production wanes, and type 2 diabetes is diagnosed. Treatment may require insulin injections for survival.

Can pomegranate juice, which has high sugar concentrations, offer health benefits for people with diabetes? Yes, although this does seem counterintuitive at first. According to a 2006 study published in the journal *Atherosclerosis,* the sugars in pomegranate juice, though similar in content to those found in other fruit juices, did not worsen blood sugar levels in the adults who consumed several ounces of pomegranate juice daily for three months. In fact, pomegranate juice *reduced* the risk of atherosclerosis.

Researchers involved in the study explain that the sugars in most juices exist in free forms, which are more likely to contribute to the problems of metabolic syndrome and atherosclerosis. The sugars in pomegranate juice, on the other hand, attach to particular antioxidants, making these sugars protective against the free-radical/inflammation cascade that leads to atherosclerosis. In the study, the consumption of pomegranate juice resulted in antioxidative effects in blood serum and on macrophages, which could contribute to healthy cardiovascular function.

In another study, pomegranate juice improved the lipid profiles of people with diabetes who had hyperlipidemia (high cholesterol). Researchers observed significant reductions in total cholesterol following daily consumption of concentrated pomegranate juice for eight weeks. They concluded that pomegranate juice may modify heart disease risk factors in those with diabetes and high cholesterol, and suggested that they might benefit from adding pomegranate juice to their diets.

HYPERLIPIDEMIA
An abnormally large amount of lipids (fats)
in the circulating blood.

In diabetes, excessive sugar in the blood can increase the stickiness of blood, making it more likely to clot and block the passage of blood through the vessels. Excess sugar may also be turned into excess fat. Even if the overall fat in the body is not increased, the fat created in the insulin-resistant state tends to collect in the abdomen, creating a condition known as abdominal obesity. Abdominal fat is highly active metabolically and is more likely to lead to hyperlipidemia and heart disease.

Most often, insulin resistance both causes and results in a surplus of overall body fat that accumulates enough to endanger a person's health. This surplus is called obesity.

Obesity

Another effect of insulin resistance lies at the root of obesity. When food containing fat, protein, or carbohydrates is eaten, the food is broken down and turned into sugars. These sugars are normally taken up into cells to fulfill the cells' energy requirements. If no immediate energy requirements exist, or if a surplus of these sugars exists, the sugars are turned into a storage molecule called glycogen, and the glycogen is stored in muscle or the liver for later use.

When the body cannot utilize glucose in a normal manner, the excess sugars that might otherwise be stored as glycogen are stored preferentially as fat. Different people can eat the same food, consume the same amount of sugars, and even engage in the same amount of activity, but only some of them become overweight. Why? The answer typically has to do with insulin resistance.

Fat stored in fat cells is not passive. Adipocytes create inflammation and increase oxidative tension by secreting special biochemical factors called cytokines. The resulting dramatic increase in the amount of inflammation and oxidation experienced throughout the body is believed to be an important link between obesity and autoimmune diseases, an enhanced risk of cancer, and heart disease.

Insulin resistance and obesity disturb the way a body stores energy at the molecular level. Certain enzymes get upregulated (their activity increases), others get downregulated (their activity decreases). The next thing you know, oxidation sneaks in along with signs of aging, cancer, and cardiovascular disease.

So, can the pomegranate offer help for the obese? A 2004 Japanese study suggests that it can. In the study, pomegranate seed oil was administered to a special kind of rat (Otsuka Long-Evans Tokushima Fatty, OLETF) that naturally develops obesity and high blood levels of fats. The OLETF rats that consumed pomegranate seed oil had lower levels of triglycerides in their livers and lower blood levels of monounsaturated fatty acid (MUFA), a major storage form of fatty acids in the body.

Punicic Acid—A Fat That Fights Obesity?

The effect of pomegranate seed oil (PSO) on decreasing the storage forms of fat that lead to obesity is believed to be related to PSO's high content of punicic acid. This is the conjugated fatty acid (meaning it has a unique configuration where unsaturated bonds alternate with saturated bonds) that makes up 65 percent of the volume of PSO.

Conjugated linoleic acids (CLAs) have promise as weight-loss aids, appearing to help boost the body's propensity toward burning stored fat for energy. CLAs have been found to aid in efforts to shed excess pounds. These molecules also have the effect of lowering insulin resistance and reducing inflammation. Research into the anti-obesity effects of punicic acid, which is quite similar in structure to CLA, is limited at this writing but promising. All conjugated fatty acids are physiologically potent anti-inflammatory agents, but punicic acid has been found to be especially potent in this regard.

Given all these positive attributes, the pomegranate fruit may be an important source of biomolecules for the fight against the many adverse effects of obesity. The greatest benefit in this regard would come from supplements incorporating elements of the whole fruit, peel, and seed included, so all of the beneficial plant chemicals would be consumed. The second-best way to reap the fruit's anti-obesity, anti-diabetes benefits would be to combine its two major fractions by consuming the arils, fresh, dried, or fermented (*see* Practical Tips and Recipes, and Resources).

Evidence of the pomegranate's many benefits for the serious problems of metabolic syndrome, obesity, and type 2 diabetes continues to mount. We look forward to future trials involving the compounds found in pomegranates for these conditions. In the meantime, you have everything to gain, and weight to lose, by adding an intelligent program of pomegranate supplementation to your diet.

7

The Most Beautiful Fruit

When it comes to exterior beauty, studies indicate that pomegranate extracts have much to offer your epidermis—the outer layer of the skin—other than its ruby juice turning your hands red. These days, pomegranate is a key ingredient in skincare and bath products. The oil from pomegranate seeds may help prevent signs of wrinkling. Pomegranate seed oil has the potential to facilitate skin repair by promoting regeneration of the outer skin layers. Topical application of products containing pomegranate has been effective in preventing sun damage. Recent studies also indicate that pomegranate extract inhibits the growth of skin tumors.

Anti-Aging Help

Though the quest for eternal youth is an ancient pastime, the demand for anti-aging products and medical treatments applied for the purpose of turning back the clock on the skin-aging process has gained momentum in the past couple of decades. Americans spend more than $12 billion each year on cosmetics and skincare products to hide or prevent the signs of aging.

What exactly is going on with our skin that would require such strenuous intervention? As it ages, skin undergoes some substantial changes:

- Skin cells divide more slowly, and the dermis—the inner layer of the skin—starts to thin

- Fat cells beneath the dermis begin to diminish

- The underlying web of elastin and collagen fibers unravels and loosens, accelerated by environmental factors, including oxygen, pollution, smoke, and sun, as well as internal triggers such as stress and bodily processes

- Skin loses its elasticity—you can see this when you press a finger into your skin and it no longer springs back to its initial position

- The glands that produce sweat and oil atrophy, diminishing the skin's protective water-lipid emulsions

- The skin retains less moisture and becomes dry and scaly

- Habitual facial expressions and small-muscle contractions cause frown lines and crow's feet to appear on facial skin

- Gravity contributes to the formation of jowls and drooping eyelids

The skin's aging process is multifaceted and happens gradually and continuously through the years. Statistics show that many men and women are doing their best to intervene. The American Society of Plastic Surgeons reports that Americans are spending a remarkable $9.4 billion annually on cosmetic plastic surgery, in spite of all the money being spent on cosmetics and beauty products. Botox treatments have increased nearly 400 percent since 2001. Other procedures, such as dermabrasion and laser skin resurfacing, are on the rise as well. Yet, these often expensive and sometimes invasive treatments aren't for everybody. Many consumers prefer a more natural approach that helps them not only to slow the signs of the passage of years, but also helps them look their best without extreme efforts to look far younger than their true age. They want products that will protect skin against damage and promote vital, glowing epidermal health.

Many of the countless anti-aging skincare products available on the market today make your skin look younger without stimulating an actual change in your skin's health or tone. Besides providing protection from the sun, the best anti-aging skin creams are *cosmeceuticals*—cosmetic products that actually induce healing or other changes in the skin cells. The active ingredients in cosmeceuticals include vitamins, especially vitamins A, C, D, and E; minerals, such as selenium and zinc; and sometimes herbal extracts or other specific antioxidants.

> **ANTIOXIDANT**
> In skin care, a substance that helps neutralize free radicals that attack cells, damage collagen and elastin, and can result in wrinkles and fine lines.

How do antioxidants combat the skin's aging process? The main goal of these antioxidants is to interfere with the process of oxidation. Everyone knows that oxygen is an essential element to life, but it can have a negative impact on skin over time. Coupled with the effects of ultraviolet (UV) rays from the sun, oxygen causes a lot of free-radical damage that shows up on skin as age spots, wrinkles, or even skin cancers. All of these changes are derived, at least in part, from oxidative cell destruction and free radical–induced tissue damage, including damage to the collagen and elastin in the skin.

You already know that antioxidants can protect the inside of your body against free-radical damage. They do so by neutralizing the free radicals that result from normal metabolism or oxidation and are accelerated by pollutants, stress, and sun. Some antioxidants prevent the damage from starting, others stop the damage while it is occurring, while still others facilitate repair after the damage has occurred. Current research into skin care shows that topically applied antioxidants can relieve—and sometimes prevent—the damaging effects of oxidation. Pomegranates are high in some of the most potent antioxidants. Pomegranate seed oil is also a wonderful skincare product in and of itself.

Pomegranates contain a higher percentage of antioxidants than any other common fruit. One antioxidant in pomegranates—ellagic acid—seems to strengthen cell membranes, making them less vulnerable to free-radical damage while preventing water loss from the cell. Ellagic acid is a particularly useful addition to skincare products.

One study found that pomegranate fruit extract (PFE), when added to skin cell cultures, inhibited the damage done by UV-A and UV-B rays. Another study, in which Dr. Lansky was a co-investigator, found that pomegranate extracts increased the synthesis of *procollagen,* a building block of skin tissue, and decreased the expression of the skin matrix metalloproteinases associated with inflammation. These kinds of investigations have caused many skincare companies to begin adding pomegranate extracts and oils to their products.

Pomegranates contain other phytochemicals—plant chemicals—that seem to provide assistance to aging skin. Pomegranates contain small amounts of estrogens identical to those made in the human body as well as the other plant estrogens mentioned in Chapters 1, 2, and 3. Estrogen plays a vital role in skin thickening, as well as in collagen and elastin replacement. After age twenty-five, estrogen production in women decreases gradually and continually throughout their lives, with a precipitous drop at menopause. This change is one major cause of skin aging in women. Replacing estrogen either orally or topically has been found to reduce the characteristic changes seen in women's skin as they age. Applied directly to the skin, estrogen creams have been found to slow thinning of skin, wrinkling, and skin discoloration in postmenopausal women. One study conducted at the University of Vienna Medical School's Department of Dermatology investigated the application of estrogen creams on the facial and neck areas of women. After six months of treatment, the skin's elasticity and firmness improved, while wrinkle depth and pore size were reduced.

This evidence points to useful roles for phytoestrogens, which mimic estrogens in the body. When consumed in the diet and applied to skin, it appears that phytoestrogens, such as those found in pomegranate seed oil, can improve the appearance and texture of the body's largest organ.

Skin care isn't just an external science. Besides taking advantage of the therapeutic benefits of pomegranate through topical application, similar benefits can be gained from ingesting the fruit. Nutritive supplements, liquid extracts, foods, and beverages containing pomegranate can help your skin from within.

Skin Repair

Studies suggest that pomegranate seed oil is a natural anti-inflammatory and anti-microbial compound. It is becoming popular in a variety of skincare formulas besides anti-aging creams. Pomegranate extract is making an appearance in medicated products designed to provide relief from, and help heal, minor skin irritations and inflammation. You can even apply a few drops of pomegranate seed oil directly to irritated skin to assist in the healing process. For any chronic or severe skin conditions, consult with your healthcare professional for appropriate treatment.

Changes in the quality of skin over time include changes not only to its appearance, but also to its ability to protect your body. Fat cells beneath the skin gradually diminish, and your inner layer of skin continues to thin as you age. Thinning skin becomes more vulnerable to injuries and damage. Also, the ability of the skin to repair itself when injured diminishes with age as wounds become slower to heal. The same properties in pomegranates that help improve the appearance of skin can also help prevent injuries to the skin as well as heal them when they occur.

Sun Protection

Pomegranate extract is showing promise as a natural agent to reduce sunlight damage—an important discovery for Western countries since the rate of skin cancer is increasing there faster than any other type of malignant disease. Skin cancer is already the most common type of cancer in the United States, with more than 1.3 million cases diagnosed each year.

> **SUN PROTECTION FACTOR, OR SPF**
> A laboratory measure of the effectiveness of a sunscreen, indicating how long a person with the sunscreen applied can be exposed to sunlight before getting burned.

In a recent laboratory study, the enhancing effect of pomegranate extract—both taken internally and applied externally—on sun protection factor (SPF) in humans was measured. Compared with lotions not containing pomegranate extract, those with pomegranate had a 20 percent higher SPF. Ingesting supplements of pomegranate extract resulted in an additional 25 percent improvement in the overall SPF of the tested products.

Skin Cancer Prevention

Besides its SPF-boosting abilities, pomegranate appears to inhibit the growth of skin tumors. This is a significant clinical finding by the American Association for Cancer Research and other well-respected research institutions.

In a South Dakota State University study, pomegranate extract was applied topically to skin tumors on mice. After five weeks, the study concluded that topical application of pomegranate seed oil inhibited growth of those tumors and the development of new tumors. In a similar study at the University of Wisconsin, researchers evaluated the anti-skin-tumor effects of pomegranate extract on mouse skin. Pomegranate extract was applied topically to some of the mice, and a strong promoter of chemically induced skin cancer was then applied to the skin of all the mice. Animals pre-treated with pomegranate extract had a 70 percent lower incidence of tumors. When tumors did develop, they were smaller than those that developed in the mice who did not receive the pomegranate extract.

When irradiated with ultraviolet light in a test tube, human cells typically undergo stress-induced inflammatory changes that can lead to cancer. In yet another study, researchers reported the results of treating cultured skin cells with pomegranate extract. Pomegranate extract dramatically inhibited those pre-carcinogenic changes in skin cells treated with the extract.

These and other studies in the cosmetics industry and beyond show that pomegranate seed oil helps invigorate the skin, reduce fine wrinkles, and soothe minor skin irritations. Whether applied topically or taken internally, the potent anti-oxidants in pomegranates help protect the skin from the free-radical damage that results from oxidation. Pomegranate extract may help prevent skin cancer. Pomegranate seed oils, extracts, and phytochemicals can be found in all the preparations below.

- Bar soap

- Bath and shower gel

- Bath salts

- Body lotion and oil

- Body scrub and polish

- Body spray

- Facial and body cleanser

- Facial cream, including moisturizing and anti-aging cream

- Hand cream

- Lip gel and gloss

- Moisturizing sunscreen

- Pomegranate seed oil for topical application

- Shampoo and conditioner

8

Today's Best Pomegranate Products and Supplements

The pomegranate—considered an exotic fruit not too long ago—has indeed gone mainstream, popping up in juices, dressings, martinis, Frappuccinos®, extracts, nutritional supplements, body lotions, and delectable dishes. Its long history of medicinal use, its many mentions in religious and spiritual texts, and a growing body of scientific research all collude to illuminate its role in promoting better health.

Now you've seen how this fruit's distinct qualities, phytochemicals, and phytohormones help your metabolic and endocrine systems to normalize. Its antioxidants seem to alleviate some of the less exhilarating changes through which aging exteriors often go. Women are finding the pomegranate useful for menopausal complaints and for the prevention of breast cancer. Men are turning to the fruit for help in their quest for better prostate health and natural function. And those concerned with their heart health are discovering that the pomegranate shows promise against cardiovascular ailments. So, why and how is this popular fruit so effective for many conditions affecting men and women, young and old?

Better Than the Sum of Its Parts?

It just may be that the potent synergy of the pomegranate's compounds contributes to—or is responsible for—the fruit's healing punch. The pomegranate boasts not only a unique flavor, but a unique biochemistry as well, containing numerous compounds considered rare in the plant world.

When the scientific and pharmaceutical communities catch wind of the health benefits from a plant or herb, researchers typically work to isolate the one ingredient responsible for the healing. As more and more bioactive compounds from the pomegranate are revealed, science mounts more research to figure out how those components of the whole food might be useful individually.

The reality is that single ingredients—whether an isolated natural ingredient from a food, or a synthetic analog made by a drug company and patented to treat a specific health condition—often do not hold the power of the synergistic activity of nutrients and phytochemicals found in a whole food. The whole is often greater than its parts in nutrition. Swallowing a pill substituting synthetic ellagic acid for the natural array of polyphenols will not provide your body with the health benefits of the whole fruit, its juice, or supplements concentrated in the natural components. This is why, when you seek out a supplement that will bring you the benefits of concentrated pomegranate, it is most sensible to seek one that contains a balance of extracts from the whole fruit, rather than single, isolated phytochemicals from pomegranate, or even less preferably, substituting synthetic ellagic acid for the real fruit components.

The potential chemopreventive effect of ellagic acid has given rise to pomegranate nutraceuticals with labels that proudly announce they are "standardized to 40 percent [or more!] ellagic acid." This is a substantially higher ellagic-acid concentration than the free ellagic acid which naturally occurs in the fruit (approximately 9 percent of total polyphenols and only 0.14 percent of total fruit). As you can see, going from 0.14 to 40 percent or more is impossible and these products are mislabeled. Some companies are unscrupulously mixing synthetic ellagic acid into their raw material. Real pomegranate extract powder containing complex compounds costs $100–$200 per kg. Synthetic ellagic acid is only $30 per kg—and it dilutes the effectiveness of the formula. It is also an *additive* and under the Dietary Supplement Health and Education Act (DSHEA) labeling laws, such products are mislabeled because added ellagic acid is a separate component, not part of the naturally occurring fruit. According to the FDA, it must be labeled clearly as a different and separate ingredient from the pomegranate.

Consumers should know that the synergy of the various pomegranate fractions and phytochemicals is more important than maximizing concentrations of any one phytochemical. The likely therapeutic chemoprevention range of ellagic acid is probably below 40 percent. It is maximized from the complexed food, not a synthetically spiked product.

The pomegranate, then, seems to offer its many benefits through the powerful synergy of its individual compounds. Many of these benefits have already been addressed in this book.

Pomegranate juice can be placed in the refrigerated section or on the shelf with other juices. However, read the label and avoid any added sugar, fructose, corn sweetener, etc. Read the Nutrition Facts label for sugar content. The naturally occurring

Herbal Remedies

As with any drug, an herbal remedy can affect how other medications or treatments work, so consult a nutritionally aware physician or other qualified healthcare professional with any concerns. To get the highest quality, be sure to buy herbal forms of pomegranate from a reputable source.

amount should be approximately 30 grams per 8 ounces of juice or 2 ounces of concentrate, or 7 grams of sugar per tablespoon of concentrate. If the sugar content is higher than this approximate amount, there is added sugar.

Concentrates are convenient and versatile. Only two ounces —six tablespoons—of concentrate is equal to a whole cup of juice. Concentrates can be mixed into other juices, milk, yogurt, diluted with water, or just swallowed like a shot of spirits. Concentrates have the advantage of making daily compliance easier, and they are also blended by manufacturers with other concentrates such as grape or blueberry.

Another issue is purity. Botanical concentrates and extracts are sometimes contaminated with lead. This is an increasing concern when materials are sourced from Eastern Europe and other regions where pollution is an issue. Accordingly, our Resources section recommends products that we know have been carefully screened to meet California's strict Proposition 65 standard requiring lead levels way below the level that could be harmful. One hundred percent lead free is impossible both because lead is naturally occurring and because of pollution. Ultra low and harmless levels of lead, however, are achievable, and we require that pomegranate products meet this standard before we recommend them. As we have not screened all products, the absence of a product on our list should not be presumed to mean it is not sufficiently pure.

See the Resources section for specific suppliers.

9

Pomegranate as a Source
of Beneficial Compounds

n the preceding pages, we have cited many examples of the use of fresh pomegranates, their juice, their seed oil, and specific synergistically prepared nutritional supplements for benefiting a wide range of health conditions. Still, though these applications may improve general health or ameliorate particular health problems, their use is not strictly medical. In other words, the fruit or its extracts are not used as pharmaceutical drugs, or medicines.

The vast field of nutritional supplements has risen up, in part, to help bridge the gap between food and medicines. Yet, for treating extreme medical problems, most physicians and perhaps even their patients, still prefer to utilize prescription *drugs* or pharmaceuticals, and this is not likely to change.

For all their status, pharmaceutical products are fraught with many disadvantages, largely owing to the deficiencies of pure chemicals compared to complex natural products. The pure chemicals generally lack the synergistic benefits and pleiotropic effects of the complex products. But because they are much easier to standardize for research purposes and to evaluate in the laboratory, pure chemicals are preferred by most medical professionals for the "treatment or prevention of disease."

Not *all* drugs, however, consist of pure chemicals, only most. In fact, one of the most commercially successful drugs of all time, Wyeth Ayerest's *Premarin*®, was and is a complex product and is therefore worthy of consideration as a model for such drugs. The name *Premarin* is a composite coming from the words "pregnant mare urine" and though more than fifty years old, it is still the world's most popular medicine prescribed for conventional hormone replacement therapy. Unlike virtually all other pharmaceuticals, it is not a single compound but a mixture derived from and only partially purified from the unappetizing source cited above. It contains at least 300 different individual chemicals. Its adherents, both patients and their physicians, prefer it simply because they believe that it "works better" than the vast array of pure compounds which constitutes its competitors.

In spite of this singular example, the American market does not presently offer any complex drugs (containing multiple compounds) derived from plants. Thankfully, though, there are a few in development. Because of the startling results we have observed in our own research with anti-cancer chemicals (i.e., finding combinations of pure chemicals more effective than single chemicals), we have chosen the path of a complex pharmaceutical as our own in our quest to develop a new compound from pomegranate for the treatment and/or prevention of human cancers.

We are currently developing a pomegranate compound called "Punisyn." Its name was derived from *puni-*, the Latin name for the pomegranate genus, and *-syn*, for the concept of synergy which accrues from the combination of specific pomegranate chemicals in carefully controlled and regulated proportions. If our initial and ongoing experimental results with Punisyn are any indication, we appear to be on the correct path. If this project succeeds, it could stimulate the development of more complex, plant-derived medicinal agents for the treatment and prevention of human disease. Individuals reading these words who have the interest and wherewithal to support our endeavor are directed to the Resources section.

Conclusion

Now you are aware that this fruit with many seeds has a diverse array of nutritional, medicinal, culinary, and cosmetic uses. The pomegranate since ancient times has held a position of importance in many cultures, with links to fertility, abundance, royalty, and righteousness.

Alongside the fruit's spiritual importance came its presence in folk medicine to treat ailments from dysentery to gum disease. Hippocrates noted the power of boiled pomegranate juice to reduce a fever.

Today, science is proving that the seeds, juice, flowers, leaves, rind, bark, and roots all have something amazing to offer. You can count on the pomegranate remaining a focus of medical and other scientific research for some time to come.

If you are unable to drink pomegranate juice because of its sugars (this may be the case if you have diabetes or are obese), a supplement containing an extract of pomegranate may be a wiser choice for you. Or, if you are interested in using a specific fraction of the pomegranate because of the research cited in this book (for example, if you would like to use pomegranate seed oil for skin care, or an extract of the whole fruit to support your passage through menopause or to protect your heart), choose one that promises a blend of synergistic ingredients rather than single, isolated chemical compounds. The websites listed in the Resources section will lead you to more information on similar supplements.

Practical Tips
and Recipes

PRACTICAL TIPS

How to Eat a Pomegranate

First, be sure to get a good, ripe specimen. The fruit should be available from September through November. A perfectly ripe pomegranate will be shiny and firm, and will feel heavy for its size. Large pomegranates are usually tastier than small ones. Tap the fruit. If it makes a metallic sound, it's ripe. Avoid fruits that look shriveled or cracked.

To remove the arils, first wash the pomegranate well, then cut the calyx out with the tip of a sharp knife. Score the outer skin in four places around the hole. Along those scores, you will be able to gently split the fruit into quarters. Tap the arils out into a bowl or plate. To avoid squirting juice all around, you can do this in a bowl of cool water; the arils will naturally separate from the peel and whitish *pericarp* (the membrane that holds the arils), both of which will float to the surface.

Some people eat each aril, seed and all. Others suck the juice from the arils and spit out the seeds. From what we know about the health value of those seeds, you would be well advised to eat at least some of them.

Use a citrus juicer to juice a halved pomegranate. You can

also make pomegranate juice inside the fruit. Simply roll the fruit around on a tabletop or between your palms, pressing hard enough to crush the arils, but not hard enough to split the peel. Then, cut out the calyx and slurp out the juice, or dribble it into a glass. The juice will oxidize if it is stored for too long. If you buy pomegranate juice from the store, it should be bright red, not brownish.

Pomegranates can be stored at room temperature. They do not continue to ripen once picked, although they may lose some of their juiciness if left out for too long. The fruit keeps well in the refrigerator for up to a month. You can freeze pomegranate arils for later use.

Using Pomegranate in Everyday Meals

- Sprinkle arils over green salad; top with orange sections and balsamic vinaigrette.

- Add arils or juice (or both) to smoothies.

- Add arils to baked goods (muffins, quickbreads) where berries are called for. They make an especially good substitute for cranberries.

- Add arils to hot cereal or yogurt.

- Make a pomegranate juice cocktail with sparkling water or lemon-lime cola: use $3/4$ water or cola and $1/4$ juice. Garnish with a slice of lime.

- Substitute pomegranate juice for citrus juice in recipes that call for it.

- Top grilled, roasted, or broiled meats with a sprinkling of arils, or with a pomegranate seed salsa.

RECIPES

SOUPS

POMEGRANATE-MISO BORSCHT SOUP

Yield: *4 servings*

3 liters spring water

$\frac{1}{4}$ cup pomegranate juice concentrate, or 1 cup fresh
pomegranate juice

1 pinch saffron

4 large organically grown beets

1 head of white or purple cabbage

4 large onions

2 large tomatoes

$\frac{1}{4}$ cup white miso, or $\frac{1}{8}$ cup *mugi* or *hatcho* miso

---

Equipment: 1 large stainless steel pot with cover

Method

Place water in pot and begin to boil. Add pomegranate juice concentrate and saffron.

Wash and cut vegetables and add to pot. Slice the beets and cabbage lengthwise to form large, very thin slices. Be sure to remove tomato stems.

Simmer at low temperature for two hours. Remove $\frac{1}{2}$ cup of boiling broth and mix with the miso in a separate cup or bowl. Add the miso mixture to the pot and turn off the burner. Allow to settle for 10 minutes before serving. Goes well with thick dark rye bread, and butter or olive oil.

Original pomegranate recipe by Ephraim Lansky, M.D.

SALADS AND SALAD DRESSINGS

POMEGRANATE CAESAR SALAD

Yield: *4 servings*

1 organic egg

1 tablespoon pomegranate juice
concentrate

$\frac{1}{4}$ cup virgin olive oil

5 cloves fresh garlic

1 small bottle anchovies in olive oil

Whole black peppercorns

1 large head romaine lettuce

1 cup fresh pomegranate arils

$\frac{1}{4}$ cup slivered blanched almonds

Equipment: One large salad bowl
Plastic lettuce spinner

Method

Crack the egg and separate the yolk. Place the egg yolk in the
bowl, along with the pomegranate juice concentrate, olive oil,
finely chopped or pressed garlic, crushed or finely chopped
anchovies, and a little freshly ground black pepper. Mix well.

Wash the lettuce well in cold water, and use salad spinner
to remove all water after washing. Break the lettuce leaves
by hand and add to the salad bowl. Toss the leaves with
the dressing. Garnish with the arils and sliced almonds.
Add additional freshly ground black pepper to taste.

Original pomegranate recipe by Ephraim Lansky, M.D.

POMEGRANATE VINEGAR

*This is easy to make and tastes wonderful
in salad dressings and marinades.*

Yield: *2$\frac{1}{2}$ cups*

1 cup pomegranate arils

2 cups white wine vinegar

Method

Sterilize a jar by boiling it for a minute, then remove it from the boiling water with tongs that have been dipped in the boiling water.

Place pomegranate seeds in the dry sterilized jar. Add white wine vinegar and seal with a tight lid.

Place the jar in a sunny spot and let stand for 8–10 days.

Strain with cheesecloth, and then pour into clean, dry bottles. You can keep this vinegar for up to six months.

SAUCES AND DIPS

POMEGRANATE SALSA

Yield: *6 servings*

2 cups pomegranate arils

1 medium-size jalapeno pepper, chopped

3–4 yellow, red, or orange bell peppers,
chopped, to taste

3–4 tablespoons cilantro

1 tablespoon sugar

1 tablespoon rice vinegar

$\frac{1}{4}$ cup pomegranate juice.

Method

Combine the first six ingredients. Mix in pomegranate juice.

FISH AND SEAFOOD

SALMON WITH POMEGRANATE SAUCE

Yield: *4 servings*

1$\frac{1}{2}$ pounds fresh salmon filets

2 tablespoons pomegranate juice
concentrate

1 lemon

1 teaspoon *umeboshi* plum vinegar,
or *shoyu* (tamari) soy sauce

1 handful cashew nuts, unsalted

1 ounce fresh ginger root

Equipment: 1 large, wide covered pot
Grater

Method

Place the filet(s) in the pot. Cover with the pomegranate juice
concentrate, lemon juice, *umeboshi* vinegar, and cashew nuts.
Grate the ginger root and spread over the fish. Cover the pot,
and simmer on a low fire for 40 minutes.

Original pomegranate recipe by Ephraim Lansky, M.D.

POULTRY

ROASTED POMEGRANATE CHICKEN

Yield: *4 servings*

$\frac{1}{4}$ cup olive oil

1 tablespoon minced garlic

1 3–4 pound chicken, quartered

1 pomegranate, halved

$\frac{1}{4}$ cup dry white wine

Juice of 1 lemon

1 tablespoon cinnamon sugar

Salt and pepper

Method

Preheat oven to 375°F. In a cup, mix oil and garlic. Brush garlic oil over chicken. Place chicken in a shallow baking dish. Drizzle any remaining oil over chicken. Bake in preheated oven for 45 minutes, basting several times with pan juices, until skin is browned and juices run clear when a thigh is pierced at the thickest part with a fork.

Remove 1 tablespoon of arils from the pomegranate. Set aside for garnish. Squeeze juice from remaining pomegranate through a sieve into a small bowl.

In a small non-reactive saucepan, mix pomegranate juice, wine, lemon juice, and cinnamon sugar. Bring to a boil over high heat. Reduce heat to low and cook 5 minutes. Season sauce with salt and pepper to taste.

Transfer roasted chicken to a serving platter and pierce each piece several times. Pour sauce over chicken. Garnish with pomegranate arils and serve at room temperature.

Recipe from: Everyday Cooking for the Jewish Home: More than 350 Delectable Recipes *by Ethel G. Hofman. New York: HarperCollins, 1997.*

MEATS

BAKED POMEGRANATE LAMB

Yield: *4 servings*

Cold water to cover

1 lamb shoulder or two lamb necks

2 cups coarse salt

8 medium onions, peeled, whole

4 heads garlic, washed, scrubbed, trimmed, optional

2 fennel bunches, quartered, optional

2 heads cabbage, quartered

1 large handful fresh or one small handful dried garden herbs
(select from parsley, sage, rosemary, thyme, or *zaatar**)

1 leek cut into 1-inch pieces, optional

$3\frac{1}{2}$ ounces pine nuts (pignolia)

2 cups dry pomegranate wine

Zaatar is an Israeli spice mixture. You can make your own with $\frac{1}{2}$ cup thyme, $\frac{1}{4}$ cup sumac (a Middle Eastern spice with a sour taste), $\frac{1}{2}$ teaspoon sea salt, and 2 tablespoons sesame seeds, all ground into a fine powder.

Equipment: Dutch oven or other closed enamel, iron, or
stainless steel cooking pot (no aluminum),
or glass or ceramic baking dish.

Oven Method

Wash the lamb well and soak it in cold water for one hour. Remove from the water and shake dry. Place on clean surface and cover with the coarse salt. Allow to sit for 18 minutes. Wash the salt off the meat, and soak in water for 5 minutes. To remove all salt, continue to wash the meat and soak again in water for 5 minutes for at least five rounds.

Place the meat in the covered pot or Dutch oven. Arrange the onions, garlic bulbs, fennel pieces, cabbage, herbs, leek, and pine nuts around it.

Pour the wine over all, cover, and bake in oven for three hours at 350°F. Serve with pressure-cooked brown rice.

Original pomegranate recipe by Ephraim Lansky, M.D.

DRINKS

POMEGRANATE-INFUSED VODKA

This is a wonderful homemade gift. In the San Francisco Chronicle, *chef-writer Dabney Gough recommends the following procedure.*

Yield: *2 cups*

1 medium pomegranate

1 medium lime

1 1/2 cups of quality vodka

Method

Remove the arils and gently crush them on a cutting board with a rolling pin, then set aside.

Cut zest from the lime peel in thin strips, being sure to avoid the bitter white pith. In a 1 1/2 quart jar, combine vodka, pomegranate arils, and lime zest.

Cover tightly, shake gently, and let sit in a dark, cool place. Shake it every few days. It should be ready after two weeks.

Strain the infused vodka into a clean bottle.

DRY POMEGRANATE WINE

Yield: *1 quart*

18 pounds of pomegranates

1/2 cup sugar, if needed

Mineral water, if needed

1 gram white wine yeast, optional

Equipment:	1 citrus juicer	1 one-gallon glass jug
	1 surgical glove	1 rubber band

Method

Wash the pomegranates well and cut them in half horizontally. Juice the fruits and collect all the juice. You should have about 1 quart at the end.

Pour the juice into the glass jug. If it is not very sweet, you may add a little sugar, but not more than half a cup. You can also add a little mineral water, but also not more than half a cup. Add the wine yeast—the type made for white wine works well. If you cannot find the wine yeast, don't use any other type. The pomegranates will find the right yeasts in the air to make it work anyway.

Turn the glove inside out, and then stretch the bottom end around the top of the bottle, securing it with a rubber band. (The glove is turned inside out to prevent powder from getting into the bottle.)

Put the jug on a shelf at room temperature. Warm temperatures will result in more rapid and facile fermentations, but cooler temperatures will result in a smoother and more subtle product. Within a few hours, you will begin to see gases accumulating inside the glove. When the gas pressure reaches a certain level, the glove will stand upright. When the glove finally reverts to its original flaccid tone, the fermentation is completed. This usually takes about ten days to two weeks. The jug can be left undisturbed for many weeks to age it further, but it should be ready to drink or cook within just 2–3 weeks. If desired, the wine can be bottled and allowed to age.

Variations

Sweet pomegranate wine. Use the above recipe. At the end of fermentation, add sugar to taste. Then add additional alcohol, preferably pomegranate spirits, but pure grain spirits will also suffice. The final product should be at least 16 percent pure alcohol; otherwise you risk refermentation.

Potassium sorbate (0.1 percent) can also be used to arrest fermentation. The wine can then be bottled and allowed to age.

Original pomegranate recipe by Ephraim Lansky, M.D.

POMEGRANATE SYRUP

Try making your own. Although grenadines are traditionally made with pomegranates, most commercially available grenadines sold in markets contain no pomegranate, just artificial flavors and colors. Homemade grenadine syrup that does contain pomegranates is great for making drinks, and is a delicious addition to sauces and desserts, such as cheesecakes, fruit pies, or ice cream.

Yield: $1\frac{1}{2}$ to 2 cups

2 large pomegranates

$\frac{2}{3}$ cup sugar

1 tablespoon lemon juice

Method

Juice the arils of two large pomegranates, either by wrapping them in a cheesecloth and squeezing them into a bowl, or by using a citrus juicer on the horizontally cut whole fruits. To include the seeds, you can also try processing the arils in a blender.

Refrigerate the juice for up to eight hours; the sediment will sink, and you will be able to ladle the clear juice off into a saucepan. Add the sugar and lemon juice. Heat, dissolving the sugar, and cook 5 minutes—long enough for the syrup to thicken and reduce. Store in the refrigerator.

DESSERT

POMEGRANATE FIGS

Yield: *4 servings*

16 large dried figs

4 cups fresh or reconstituted
pomegranate juice

Equipment: Non-aluminum saucepan with cover.
Heat diffuser or asbestos pad.

Method

Inspect the figs carefully and rinse in cold water. Place in the saucepan with enough pomegranate juice to cover and a little more. Cover and place on a burner with the heat diffuser under the pot. Simmer on a very low fire for five hours or until most of the liquid is absorbed into the figs. Additional juice can be added if the process seems to be going too fast.

Once the cooking has been completed, the fruit can be enjoyed warm with heavy cream or tahini sauce. Alternatively, the moist figs can be placed in a tightly sealed glass jar with a little of the sauce and kept practically indefinitely in the refrigerator. Excellent!

Original pomegranate recipe by Ephraim Lansky, M.D.

Resources

Jarrow Formulas®, Inc.

1824 S. Robertson Blvd.
Los Angeles, CA 90035
Phone: 310-204-6936
Toll-free: 800-726-0886
www.jarrow.com

Dietary supplements, including encapsulated pomegranate formulations and pomegranate juice concentrate, and pomegranate plus berry juice concentrate.

Products:

PomeGreat™—Pomegranate Juice Concentrate (12 and 24 fluid ounces)

PomeGreat™—Blend of Pomegranate, Grape and Blueberry Juice Concentrate

PomGuard™ (400 mg per capsule/60 capsules)—Unique blend of fermented Israel Wonderful pomegranate juice, seed meal, and aqueous extracts of peel and leaf

Pomegranate Health

439 Monroe Avenue, Suite 130
Rochester, NY 14607
Phone: 585-777-4090
Toll-free: 800-661-5176
www.pomhealth.com

Pomegranate dietary supplements, skin care products, bulk ingredients, and information.

Pom Wonderful
11444 W. Olympic Blvd.
Los Angeles, CA 90064
Phone: 310-966-5863
www.pomwonderful.com
Pomegranate juice products.

Rimonest Ltd.
1 Hadekalim Street
POB 9945
Haifa, Israel
Phone: 972-4-864-5011
www.rimonest.com

Pomegranate science, patents, consulting, information, and specialty products including fermented pomegranate juice concentrate and pomegranate seed oil.

Pomegranate Research Support

Anyone wishing to learn more and help support ongoing cancer research involving pomegranate extracts is encouraged to contact the authors.

Ephraim P. Lansky, M.D.
Punisyn Pharmaceuticals,
  Ltd.
POB 9945
Haifa, Israel
www.punisyn.com

Robert A. Newman, Ph.D.
Pharmaceutical Development
  Center
University of Texas M.D.
  Anderson Cancer Center
1515 Holcombe Blvd.
Houston, TX 77030
www.mdanderson.org

References

Afaq, F., Saleem, M., Krueger, C.G., et al. "Anthocyanin- and hydrolyzable tannin–rich pomegranate fruit extract modulates MAPK and NF-kappaB pathways and inhibits skin tumorigenesis in CD-1 mice." *International Journal of Cancer* 113:3 (January 2005): 423–433.

Ahmed, S., Wang, N., Hafeez, B.B., et al. "*Punica granatum L.* extract inhibits IL-1 beta–induced expression of matrix metalloproteinases by inhibiting the activation of MAP kinases and NF-kappaB in human chondrocytes in vitro." *Journal of Nutrition* 135:9 (September 2005): 2096–2102.

Albrecht, M., Jiang, W., Kumi-Diaka, J., et al. "Pomegranate extracts potently suppress proliferation, xenograft growth, and invasion of human prostate cancer cells." *Journal of Medicinal Foods* 7:3 (Fall 2004): 274–283.

Arao, K., Wang, Y.M., Inoue, N., et al. "Dietary effect of pomegranate seed oil rich in 9cis, 11trans, 13cis conjugated linolenic acid on lipid metabolism in obese, hyperlipidemic OLETF Rats." *Lipids in Health and Disease* 3:24 (November 2004): 476–511.

Aslam, M.N., Lansky, E.P., Varani, J. "Pomegranate as a cosmeceutical source: Pomegranate fractions promote proliferation and procollagen synthesis and inhibit matrix metalloproteinase production in human skin cells." *Journal of Ethnopharmacology* 103:3 (February 2006): 311–318.

Aviram, M., Dornfeld, L. "Pomegranate juice consumption inhibits serum angiotensin converting enzyme activity and reduces systolic blood pressure." *Atherosclerosis* 158:1 (September 2001): 195–198.

Aviram, M., Dornfeld, L., Rosenblat, M., et al. "Pomegranate juice consumption reduces oxidative stress, atherogenic modifications to LDL, and platelet aggregation: Studies in human and in atherosclerotic apolipoprotein e–deficient mice." *American Journal of Clinical Nutrition* 71:5 (May 2000): 1062–1076.

Aviram, M., Rosenblat, M., Gaitini, D., et al. "Pomegranate juice consumption for three years by patients with carotid artery stenosis reduces common carotid intima-media thickness, blood pressure, and LDL oxidation." *American Journal of Clinical Nutrition* 23:3 (June 2004): 423–433.

Azadzoi, K.M., Schulman, R.N., Aviram, M., Siroky, M.B. "Oxidative stress in arteriogenic erectile dysfunction: prophylactic role of antioxidants." *Journal of Urology* 174:1 (July 2005): 386–393.

Barch, D.H., Rundhaugen, L.M. "Ellagic acid induces NAD(P)H: quinone reductase through activation of the antioxidant responsive element of the rat NAD(p)H:quinone reductase gene." *Carcinogenesis* 15:9 (September 1994): 2065–2068.

Braga, L.C., Leite, A.A., Xavier, K.G., et al. "Synergic interaction between pomegranate extract and antibiotics against *Staphylococcus aureus*." *Canadian Journal of Microbiology* 51:7 (July 2005): 541–547.

Bryant, R. "Pomegranate extract shows promise in boosting sun protection: Fruit has a high polyphenol content." *Dermatology Times* (April 1, 2004).

De Nigris, F., Williams-Ignarro, S., Lerman, L.O., et al. "Beneficial effects of pomegranate juice on oxidation-sensitive genes and eNos activity at sites of perturbed shear-stress." *Proceedings of the National Academy of Sciences* 102:13 (2005): 4896–4901.

Esmaillzadeh, A., Tahbaz, F., Gaieni, I., et al. "Concentrated pomegranate juice improves lipid profiles in diabetic patients with hyperlipidemia." *Journal of Medicinal Food* 7:3 (Fall 2004): 305–308.

"Fruit Facts: Pomegranate." California Rare Fruit Growers, Inc., 1997. www.crfg.org/pubs/ff/pomegranate.html.

"Fruit of the Month: Pomegranate." U.S. Department of Health and Human Services, Centers for Disease Control and Prevention. www.5aday.gov/month/pomegranate.html.

Gough, Dabney. "Do-it-yourself flavored vodka." *San Francisco Chronicle* (November 24, 2006). http://sfgate.com/cg-bin/article. cgi?f=/c/a/2006/1124/WIGLBMHNAA1.DTL.

Greenberg, A.S., Obin, M.S. "Obesity and the role of adipose tissue in inflammation and metabolism." *American Journal of Clinical Nutrition* 83:2 (February 2006): 461S–465S.

Hartman, R.E., Shah, A., Fagan, A.M., et al. "Pomegranate juice decreases amyloid load and improves behavior in a mouse model of Alzheimer's disease." *Neurobiology of Disease* 24:3 (September 2006): 506–515.

Hora, J.J., Maydew, E.R., Lansky, E.P., et al. "Chemopreventive effects of pomegranate seed oil on skin tumor development in CD1 mice." *Journal of Medicinal Food* 6:3 (October 2003): 157–161.

Kaplan, M., Hayek, T., Raz, A., et al. "Pomegranate juice supplementation to atherosclerotic mice reduces macrophage lipid peroxidation, cellular cholesterol accumulation and development of atherosclerosis." *American Journal of Clinical Nutrition* 131:8 (August 2001): 2082–2089.

Kardinaal, A.F., Morton, M.S., Bruggeman-Rotgans, I.E., et al. "Phytoestrogen excretion and rate of bone loss in postmenopausal women." *European Journal of Clinical Nutrition* 52:11 (1998): 850–855.

Katz, S.R., Newman, R.A., Lansky, E.P. "*Punica granatum*: Heuristic treatment for diabetes mellitus." Journal of Medicinal Food (In Press).

Kaur, G., Jabbar, Z., Athar, M., et al. "*Punica granatum* (pomegranate) flower extract possesses potent antioxidant activity and abrogates Fe-NTA induced hepatotoxicity in mice." *Food and Chemical Toxicology* 44:7 (July 2006): 984–992.

Kawaii, S., Lansky, E.L. "Differentiation-promoting activity of pomegranate (*Punica granatum*) fruit extracts in HL-60 human promyelocytic leukemia cells." *Journal of Medicinal Food* 7:1 (April 2004): 13–18.

Kim, M.K., Chung, B.C., Yu, W.V., et al. "Relationships of urinary phyto-oestrogen excretion to bone mineral density in postmenopausal women." *Clinical Endocrinology (Oxford)* 56:3 (2002): 321–328,.

Kim, N.D., Mehta, R., Yu, W., et al. "Chemopreventive and adjuvant therapeutic potential of pomegranate (*Punica granatum*) for human breast cancer." *Breast Cancer Research and Treatment.* 71:3 (February 2002): 203–217.

Langley, P. "Why a pomegranate?" *British Medical Journal* 321:7269 (November 2000): 1153–1154.

Lansky, E.P. "Beware of pomegranates bearing 40 percent ellagic acid." *Journal of Medicinal Food* 9:1 (Spring 2006): 119–122.

Lansky, E.P., Harrison, G., Froom, P., et al. "Pomegranate (*Punica granatum*) pure chemicals show possible synergistic inhibition of human PC-3 prostate cancer cell invasion across Matrigel." *Investigational New Drugs* 23:4 (August 2005): 379.

Lansky, E.P., Jiang, W., Huanbiao, M., et al. "Possible synergistic prostate cancer suppression by anatomically discrete pomegranate fractions." *Investigational New Drugs* 23:1 (December 2004): 11–20.

Lansky, E.P., Newman, R.A.. *"Punica granatum* (pomegranate) and its potential in the prevention and treatment of inflammation and cancer." *Journal of Ethnopharmacology* 109 (2007): 177–206.

Lansky, E.P., Shubert, S., Neeman, I. "Pharmacological and therapeutic properties of pomegranate." In Melgarejo-Moreno, P., Martínez-Nicolás, J.J., Martínez-Tomé, J. (eds.). *Production, Processing and Marketing of Pomegranate in the Mediterranean Region: Advances in Research and Technology.* Zaragoza: CIHEAM-IAMZ, 2000, 231–235.

Lansky, E.P., Von Hoff, D.D. "Complex and simple." *Leukemia Research* 29 (2005): 601–602.

Loren, D.J., Seeram, N.P., Schulman, R.N., et al. "Maternal dietary supplementation with pomegranate juice is neuroprotective in an animal model of neonatal hypoxic-ischemic brain injury." *Pediatric Research* 57:6 (June 2005): 858–864.

Lempert, Phil. "Pomegranate juice steps up to the plate." *Facts, Figures, and the Future* (June 13, 2005). www.factsfiguresfuture. com/archive/june_2005.htm.

Libby, P., Ridker, P.M., Maseri, A. "Inflammation and atherosclerosis." *Circulation* 105 (2002): 1135.

Malik, A., Afaq, F., Sarfaraz, S., et al. "Pomegranate fruit juice for chemoprevention and chemotherapy of prostate cancer." *Proceedings of the National Academy of Sciences* 102:41 (October 2005): 14813–14818.

McLean, P.D. *A Triune Concept of the Brain and Behavior.* Toronto, Canada: University of Toronto Press, 1973.

Mehta, R., Lansky, E.P. "Breast cancer chemopreventive properties of pomegranate (*Punica granatum*) fruit extracts in a mouse mammary organ culture." *European Journal of Cancer Prevention* 13:4 (August 2004): 345–348.

Mori-Okamoto, J., Otawara-Hamamoto, Y., Yamato, H., et al. "Pomegranate extract improves a depressive state and bone properties in menopausal syndrome model ovariectomized mice." *Journal of Ethnopharmacology* 92:1 (May 2004): 93–101.

Narayanan, B.A., Geoffroy, O., Willingham, M.C., et al. "P53/p21(WAF1/CIP1) expression and its possible role in G1 arrest and apoptosis in ellagic acid treated cancer cells." *Cancer Letters* 136:2 (March 1999): 215–221.

"Organic Farmers' Market Report: Ruby Red Pomegranates." OrganicAuthority.com. www.organicauthority.com/organic_food/farmers_market_report_1_12.html.

Pantuck, A.J., Leppert, J.T., Zomorodian, N., et al. "Phase II study of pomegranate juice for men with rising prostate-specific antigen following surgery or radiation for prostate cancer." *Clinical Cancer Research* 12:13 (July 2006): 4018–4026.

"Pomegranate." The Fruit Institute. www.fruitinstitute.org/pomegranate.htm.

Roberts, R.O., Jacobson, D.J., Girman, C.J., et al. "A population-based study of daily nonsteroidal anti-inflammatory drug use and prostate cancer." *Mayo Clinic Proceedings* 77:3 (March 2002): 219–225.

Rosenblat, M., Hayek, T., Aviram, M. "Anti-oxidative effects of pomegranate juice (PJ) consumption by diabetic patients on serum and on macrophages." *Atherosclerosis* 187:2 (August 2006): 363–371.

Schmidt, J.B., Binder, M., Demschik, G., et al. "Treatment of skin aging with topical estrogens." *International Journal of Dermatology* 35:9 (September 1996): 669–674.

Schubert, S.Y., Lansky, E.P., Neeman, I. "Antioxidant and eicosanoid enzyme inhibition properties of pomegranate seed oil and fermented juice flavonoids." *Journal of Ethnopharmacology* 66:1 (July 1999): 11–17.

Schwartz, A. "The Seeds of a Cure?" *Jerusalem Report*. Denver, CO: Denver Naturopathic Clinic, January 2002. www.denvernaturopathic.com/news/jerusalem.html.

Sumner, M.D., Elliott-Eller, M., Weidner, G., et al. "Effects of pomegranate juice consumption on myocardial perfusion in patients with coronary heart disease." *American Journal of Cardiology* 96:6 (September 2005): 810–814.

Syed, D.N., Malik, A., Hadi, N., et al. "Photochemopreventive effect of pomegranate fruit extract on UVA-mediated activation of cellular pathways in normal human epidermal keratinocytes." *Photochemistry and Photobiology* 82:2 (March-April 2006): 398–405.

Thanos, J., Cotterchio, M., Boucher, B.A., et al. "Adolescent dietary phytoestrogen intake and breast cancer risk (Canada)." *Cancer Causes and Control* 17:10 (December 2006): 1251–1261.

Toi, M., Bando, H., Ramachandran, C., et al. "Preliminary studies on the anti-angiogenic potential of pomegranate fractions *in vitro* and *in vivo*." *Angiogenesis* 6:2 (2003): 121–128.

Tous, J., Ferguson, L. "Mediterranean fruits." In Janick, J. (ed.). *Progress in New Crops*. Arlington, VA: ASHS Press, 1996, 416–430.

Index

About the Authors

Robert A. Newman, M.S., Ph.D., received graduate training at the University of Connecticut, and postgraduate training in pharmacology and toxicology at the University of Georgia Medical School, the University of Vermont School of Medicine, and Stanford University. For the past twenty-two years, he has been a faculty member at the University of Texas M.D. Anderson Cancer Center in Houston, and currently serves there as a Professor of Cancer Medicine in the Department of Experimental Therapeutics. He also is the Director of the MDACC Pharmaceutical Development Center. He has published over 250 scientific articles dealing with various aspects of anti-cancer drug development and mechanisms of action.

Dr. Newman's current interests include development of novel agents for the prevention and treatment of malignant disease and the relationship of inflammation to disease progression. Recently, he has explored the use of herbal and plant-based medicinal products that serve to specifically reduce inflammation. These products include selected extracts derived from fig, oleander, pomegranate, and specific Chinese plants. He is affiliated with Punisyn Pharmaceuticals where he works closely with Dr. Ephraim Lansky in the development and testing of a prototype pomegranate product currently being evaluated for the prevention of human breast cancer.

Ephraim P. Lansky, M.D., completed his medical training at the University of Pennsylvania School of Medicine and his internship in medicine and psychiatry at Pennsylvania Hospital. Both institutions were founded by Benjamin Franklin in Philadelphia. For the past twenty-three years, Dr. Lansky has practiced general Complementary and Alternative Medicine (CAM), and has completed additional advanced clinical education and certification in acupuncture, classical homeopathy, hypnosis, medical herbology, and emergency medicine. He has been intensively researching the pomegranate as a medicinal article for the past fifteen years, and has published fourteen peer-reviewed scientific papers on this subject, with special focus on the pomegranate's anti-cancer, anti-inflammatory, antioxidant, and estrogenic actions. He is also the founder and Chairman of Rimonest Ltd., a biotechnology company dedicated to developing medicinal and health products from the pomegranate. Through Rimonest's new subsidiary, Punisyn Pharmaceuticals, Ltd., he is collaborating closely with Professor Robert A. Newman in the development and testing of a complex pomegranate medication for the treatment and/or prevention of human cancers, especially of the breast and prostate. Dr. Lansky lives and works in Haifa, Israel.

Melissa Lynn Block, M.Ed., is a writer and editor who specializes in health and medical titles. Her company, *ideokinesis,* helps authors bring their research, ideas, and experience to life on the printed page, in the form of books, articles, newsletters, Web content, or other print media. She has authored, co-authored, contributed to, and edited more than a dozen books, and can be contacted at ideokinesis@verizon.net.